Paediatric Cases for
Postgraduate Examinations

Titles in the series

Paediatric cases for postgraduate examinations

Simon Attard-Montalto MB ChB, MRCP, DCH
Lecturer in Paediatric Oncology
St Bartholomew's Hospital, London

Vaskar Saha MBBS, MD, DCH
Senior Registrar in Paediatric Oncology
St Bartholomew's Hospital, London

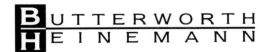

To our parents

Butterworth-Heinemann Ltd
Linacre House, Jordan Hill, Oxford OX2 8DP

ᘓ A member of the Reed Elsevier plc group

OXFORD   LONDON   BOSTON
MUNICH   NEW DELHI   SINGAPORE   SYDNEY
TOKYO   TORONTO   WELLINGTON

First published 1994
Reprinted 1995

British Library Cataloguing in Publication Data
Attard-Montalto, Simon
  Paediatric Cases for Postgraduate
  Examinations
  I. Title II. Saha, Vaskar
  618.920076

ISBN 0 7506 2096 X

Typeset by BC Typesetting, Warmley, Bristol BS15 5YD
Printed and bound in Great Britain by
Biddles Ltd, Guildford and King's Lynn

Contents

Foreword

Never in the history of medical examination conflict has so much been expected in such a short time. We now expect our juniors to have immense experience and pass examinations before they can possibly have been exposed to the very clinical cases onto which they could hang their theoretical knowledge. The only way that they can arm themselves adequately for the skirmish with examiners is to pick the brains of those who have accumulated experience but who are not too far removed from knowing what is truly required for the examination. Junior staff rounds and informal membership teaching demonstrated to the authors of this excellent tome that there was a real need for a compilation of the case reports which they had used in their own teaching. Using the case report format, Simon and Vaskar share their outstanding experience with candidates who also gain from the authors' knowledge and advice on answering one of the more testing aspects of postgraduate examinations, namely the 'grey case'.

Professor Tim Eden
Academic Department of Paediatric Oncology
St. Bartholomew's Hospital, London

Preface

Repeated practice is often the mainstay of revision for any examination. This is certainly true with regards to the section on case presentations in paediatric postgraduate examinations. Although some excellent books on paediatric case presentations have now been published, the number is small and the supply rapidly exhausted by the enterprising candidate! This compilation was initially designed as an informal *aide memoire*. However, the encouragement and enthusiasm shown by prospective candidates convinced us to publish this series in book form.

All the cases cited in this book are based on true patients, though some have been modified to suit the general format of the written examinations. The cases cover a broad spectrum of paediatrics, and although some may represent rather unusual conditions, we have tried to ensure that they are representative of the questions set in the examinations. The book has been designed primarily for candidates sitting the Membership of the Royal College of Physicians (MRCP) part II examination in paediatrics. However, the material covered should prove useful to those candidates taking other examinations, and to all those with an interest in clinical and academic paediatrics. We hope that those who read this book will enjoy the challenge posed by these cases.

List of abbreviations

ACTH	adrenocorticotrophic hormone
ALT	alanine transaminase
AST	aspartate transaminase
Ca^{2+}	calcium
Cl^-	chloride
CPK	creatinine phosphokinase
CRP	C-reactive protein
CSF	cerebrospinal fluid
CT	computerized tomogram
(°C)	degrees Celcius
ECG	electrocardiogram
ECHO	echocardiogram
EEG	electroencephalogram
EMG	electromyogram
ENT	ears, nose and throat
ESR	erythrocyte sedimentation rate
EUA	examination under anaesthesia
FDP	fibrin degradation products
FSH	follicle stimulating hormone
γGT	γ-glutamyl transpeptidase
GH	growth hormone
GP	general practitioner
Hb	haemoglobin
HCO_3^-	bicarbonate
Ig	immunoglobulin
K^+	potassium
KPPT	kaolin partial prothrombin time
LDH	lactate dehydrogenase
LFT	liver function tests
MCH	mean cell haemoglobin
MCHC	mean cell haemoglobin concentration
MCV	mean cell volume
Mg^{2+}	magnesium

MRI	magnetic resonance imaging
Na^+	sodium
PO_4^{3-}	phosphate
PT	prothrombin time
T_4	thyroxine
TPN	total parenteral nutrition
TSH	thyroid stimulating hormone
TT	thrombin time

How to use this book

Achieving a maximum score in the 'grey cases' will depend on the correct identification of the most important features in the history, examination and investigations, and putting these together in order to result in the best or the 'best fit' diagnosis.

Each question should be read twice over. Highlight the main points from the history and consider any features which you think may be relevant to the case, but which may not have been provided. Assess the physical signs in a similar manner, noting both the positive and negative (or omitted) findings. You should, at this stage, formulate a 'working differential diagnosis' and ask yourself the question 'what investigations are indicated?' Then review the investigative results provided, remembering that some of these results may be superfluous, whilst some other vital information may have been withheld. Consider whether you are now able to make a definitive diagnosis. If not (and indeed a definitive diagnosis may not be possible), consider your list of options and try to determine which would best explain the clinical and investigative scenario.

Even in particularly 'grey' cases where no clear diagnosis springs to mind, many of the questions will relate to practical issues in the patients' management, and by applying a simple 'common sense' approach, it is still possible to obtain a good score. It is often useful to consider how *you* would manage the case as the paediatric registrar seeing the patient for the first time!

The marks allocated to the answers have been 'weighted' so that maximum points have been awarded for the answers that best explain all aspects of the case. Fewer points have been allocated for those suggestions which, although reasonable, do not make up the ideal answer. The maximum score for each question is 10 but a good score may still be possible even if the precise diagnosis is incorrect. Furthermore, each question has been allocated an overall grade: Easy, Average or Hard. This grading system has been determined by several groups of prospective candidates who were asked to tackle the questions, and should only be used *as a guide* to enable you to assess your own performance.

A brief discussion follows the list of answers to each case. We have attempted to illustrate the key features in the case and why we would have decided on a particular answer as opposed to another. We have tried to emphasise the importance of the identification and interpretation of clinical symptoms and signs, and the relevance of the investigations provided. The discussion is not intended as an exhaustive review of each condition. Furthermore, we have limited references to a minimum, and have cited only review articles and excerpts from journals and textbooks which we have found useful and which are commonly available to postgraduate students.

Case presentations and questions

Case 1

A 10-month-old infant presented with a 3 week history of irritability and abdominal distension. He was born at term weighing 4.2 kg and apart from transient, asymptomatic hypoglycaemic episodes within the first 72 hours of life, he had been well.

He plotted above the 90th centile for length and weight, and was found to be miserable and pale with an asymmetric firm right sided abdominal swelling. Distended, superficial veins tracked towards a large umbilical hernia.

Investigations

Hb, 8.9 g/dl
total white cell count, $17 \times 10^9/l$
platelets, $932 \times 10^9/l$
urinalysis, no abnormality detected

Questions

1. What two investigations would best help to confirm a diagnosis?
2. What is the underlying condition?

Case 2

A girl presented at the age of 3 years with excessive thirst and polyuria. The blood glucose was normal. A diagnosis of diabetes insipidus was made and she was treated with regular desamino arginine vasopressin (DDAVP) pernasally. Her control was always difficult and deteriorated as she got older, necessitating several hospital admissions. Her behaviour was a major problem but her mother was devoted and accompanied her on each admission, administered the DDAVP and checked the urine specimens.

By the age of 8 years her weight was on the 3rd centile, height 40th centile and urine osmolality around 250 mmol/kg with a serum Na^+ level of 140 mmol/l, K^+ 4 mmol/l, urea 4 mmol/l and Ca^{2+} 2.2 mmol/l. During an admission to try and improve her control, the mother had to attend to a sudden bereavement in the family. This resulted in the child having a tantrum and refusing all medication. That evening the serum osmolality was found to be 295 mmol/kg and urine 420 mmol/kg.

Questions

1. What is the diagnosis?
2. How would you confirm this?

Case 3

A 5-month-old male infant presented with a 2 week history of a fever, cough and irritability. He was treated by the GP for conjunctivitis with amoxycillin. The symptoms did not improve, and over the following 3 days he developed a patchy, irregular rash over the cheeks and trunk and was brought to casualty by his worried mother.

On examination the cervical lymph nodes were enlarged, and the conjunctivae, gums, and fauces injected. He had flushed peripheries and a widespread macular-papular erythematous rash.

Investigations

Hb, 7.6 g/dl
total white cell count, $21 \times 10^9/l$
Na^+, 135 mmol/l
K^+, 5 mmol/l
urea, 8.2 mmol/l
Ca^{2+}, 2.3 mmol/l
creatinine, 76 mmol/l
glucose, 6.5 mmol/l

Three days after admission he became pale and breathless. He cried incessantly, was totally inconsolable and slept poorly.

Questions

1. What is the diagnosis?
2. What other investigations would be helpful on admission?
3. What complication may have occurred 3 days after admission?
4. What further investigations were indicated on day 3?
5. What treatment would be appropriate?

Case 4

A twelve-year-old boy from Pakistan was visiting his father, a post-graduate student studying in the United Kingdom. Shortly after his arrival he developed a fever, general lethargy and headaches. The high temperature persisted and, after 3 days of fever, he was taken to the local casualty department. He had mild cervical lymphadenopathy, a palpable spleen 1 cm below the costal margin, and a few non-specific spots on the abdomen. Despite intravenous ampicillin for 3 days he remained unwell with a striking temperature with spikes up to 40°C several times a day, and developed loose stools.

Investigations

Hb, 8.4 g/dl
MCV, 75 fl
MCH, 26 pg
MCHC, 32 g/dl
total white cell count, $2 \times 10^9/l$
platelets, $270 \times 10^9/l$

Questions

1. What other investigations are necessary?
2. What are the two most likely diagnoses?
3. Outline the management of this patient?

Case 5

An 8-year-old caucasian boy was admitted following a 7 day history of a cough, a high temperature and abdominal pain. On examination he was pale, icteric with injected tonsils, and had a tender abdominal mass below the left costal margin.

Investigations

Hb, 4.2 g/dl
MCV, 60 fl
total white cell count, $1.1 \times 10^9/l$
neutrophils, $0.6 \times 10^9/l$
platelets, $85 \times 10^9/l$
reticulocytes, 2%
direct Coombs' test, negative
total bilirubin, 110 μmol/l
unconjugated bilirubin, 95 μmol/l
urinalysis, no abnormality detected

Questions

1. What is the diagnosis?
2. What investigations would help to confirm this?
3. What probable complication has arisen?

Case 6

A male infant was born at 36 weeks' gestation to an 18-year-old primigravida after a difficult labour. He weighed 2.7 kg, and the Apgar score was 5 at 1 min and 7 at 5 min. He required headbox oxygen for a few minutes and was discharged home after a normal examination on day five.

He presented aged 7 days with a history of poor feeding and recent vomiting. He was pale, grey, poorly perfused with a respiratory rate of 83 breaths per minute, a pulse of 175 beats per minute and 4 cm hepatomegaly.

Investigations

Hb, 10 g/dl
total white cell count, 16×10^9/l
platelets, 193×10^9/l
glucose, 1.4 mmol/l
pH, 7.22
P_{CO_2}, 4 kPa
P_{O_2}, 5.7 kPa
base deficit, 9 (in air)
chest X-ray: heart not enlarged, widespread, diffuse shadowing in
    overexpanded lungs
ECG, axis+165°; right ventricular dominance

Questions

1. What investigations were indicated on admission?
2. What therapeutic measures were indicated?
3. What was the diagnosis?

Case 7

A neonate was born at 29 weeks' gestation to a diabetic mother,
weighing 1.3 kg. The Apgar score was 3 at 1 min and 4 at 5 min after
a difficult intubation. She was stabilized on pressures of 20/3, 50
breaths per minute and 45% oxygen, and an umbilical arterial
catheter was inserted. She received vitamin K, 0.5 mg intramuscu-
larly, shortly after birth.

Investigations

Hb, 12 g/dl
total white cell count, 10×10^9/l
platelets, 70×10^9/l
Na^+, 140 mmol/l
K^+, 4.8 mmol/l
glucose (BM stix), <1
pH, 7.05
P_{CO_2}, 7.8
P_{O_2}, 9
base deficit, 6
chest X-ray: bilateral reticular shadowing and air bronchogram

She had been improving at 83 hours of age when the oxygen saturation dropped suddenly from 90 to 62%, and the mean BP fell from 28 to 15 mmHg. She required resuscitation with plasma and increased ventilatory support.

Investigations

Hb, 7.5 g/dl
total white cell count, $13 \times 10^9/l$
platelets, $40 \times 10^9/l$
PT, 23 s (control, 12 s)
KPPT, 76 s (control, 25 s)
TT, 20 s (control 10 s)
pH, 7.21
P_{CO_2}, 4.9
P_{O_2}, 6.6
base deficit, 16
Na^+, 122 mmol/l
K^+, 7.3 mmol/l
urea, 9 mmol/l
blood glucose, 0.2 mmol/l
cranial ultrasound scan showed mild ventricular dilatation

Despite all efforts she remained severely hypotensive and hypoglycaemic and died 2 days later.

Questions

1. What immediate steps were indicated at birth?
2. What urgent investigations would you carry out after the emergency at 83 hours?
3. Name three therapeutic measures required at this time.
4. What was the cause of her collapse?

Case 8

A 9-year-old boy presented to the outpatients department with a 2 month history of recurrent left sided abdominal pain prior to micturition. Usually stoic, he cried for half an hour during each episode but was fine afterwards. He plotted on the 5th centile for height and weight and had no abnormal signs on physical examination. The BP was 106/70 mmHg.

Investigations

Hb, 9.5 g/dl
MCV, 72 fl
total white cell count, 15×10^9/l
platelets, 255×10^9/l
Na^+, 143 mmol/l
K^+, 4.2 mmol/l
urea, 6 mmol/l
creatinine, 50 mmol/l
Ca^{2+}, 2.7 mmol/l
phosphate, 1.4 mmol/l
serum iron, 7.1 μmol/l
total iron binding capacity, 98 μmol/l
urinalysis, red cells 3+; protein 2+

Question

1. How would you investigate this child?

Case 9

A 13-year-old boy had been followed up by his GP for 6 months. He had been troubled with intermittent fevers, an unproductive cough and occasional wheezing. During this period he had been treated with beta agonists and inhaled steroids with little change in his symptoms. He appeared to take a well balanced diet and did not suffer with any bowel problems. He was referred for a specialist opinion when his cough had become particularly troublesome and occasionally productive of small amounts of blood streaked sputum. At this point he had also started to complain of breathlessness on exertion and generalized tiredness.

Investigations

Hb, 7.4 g/dl
total white cell count, 16×10^9/l

platelets, $235 \times 10^9/l$
MCV, 68 fl
MCH, 19 pg
MCHC, 28 g/dl
ESR, 15 mm in the first hour
peak flow, 390 l/min (expected 330–500 l/min)
total lung capacity, 3.96 l (expected, 3.98 – 5.65 l)
vital capacity, 2.81 l (expected 2.98–4.45 l)
residual capacity, 1.3 l (expected 0.8 – 1.1 l)
forced expiratory volume in 1 s, 1.89 l (expected 2.45–3.72 l)
diffusion capacity of CO (T_LCO), 5.3 mmol/min/kPa (expected 6.9–10.4 mmol/min/kPa)
diffusion capacity per unit lung volume (KCO), 1.2 mmol/min/kPa/l (expected 1.68–2.53 mmol/min/kPa/l)
multiple sputum cultures, negative
chest X-ray: bilateral, fine, diffuse shadowing

Questions

1. What is the diagnosis?
2. How would you treat this child?

Case 10

An 8-year-old mentally retarded, partially deaf girl was admitted to the paediatric psychiatric ward for control of her difficult behaviour. Her parents were cousins and had had an arranged marriage. Their relationship was passing through a stormy phase and they were both finding their daughter's behaviour very hard to cope with.

She plotted on the 90th centile for weight and 40th centile for height, had rather coarse, hirsute features, a short, thick neck, and 4 cm hepatomegaly. X-rays of her hands showed wide metacarpals.

Questions

1. What is the diagnosis?
2. What investigations would confirm the diagnosis?
3. List the main aspects of this girl's management.

Case 11

A healthy 27-year-old primigravida was delivered of a baby girl weighing 3.0 kg at 36 weeks' gestation, after a pregnancy complicated with polyhydramnios. Several prenatal ultrasound scans had revealed no physical abnormality in the fetus. Delivery was by difficult ventouse extraction after several decelerations in the fetal heart rate during the final stages. The infant had passed meconium prior to the delivery and had Apgar scores of 2 at 1 min, and 4 at 5 min. She was ventilated and an arterial blood gas at 20 min showed a pH of 7.27, P_{O_2} 35 kPa, P_{CO_2} 4.7 kPa, and a base deficit of 4.7 in 50% oxygen. A chest X-ray showed slight streaky shadowing in the right mid-zone.

She was rapidly weaned down on the ventilator settings over 24 hours, to a rate of 10 breaths per minute, and pressures of 16/2 in air. At 36 hours she was extubated and nursed in 30% head-box oxygen, but the oxygen requirements rose over the next 12 hours: in 70% oxygen, with a respiratory rate of 55 breaths per minute, the arterial blood gas showed a pH of 7.12, P_{O_2} 15 kPa, P_{O_2} 8.2 kPa, and base deficit of 9. A chest X-ray showed atelectasis in the right mid-zone, and a cranial ultrasound scan showed a grade I haemorrhage on the left.

She was reventilated for 3 days, then extubated and feeds were commenced by nasogastric tube after 24 hours. However, she remained lethargic with a weak cry, poor sucking reflex and the large gastric aspirates persisted. On examination she was areflexic. Oxygen requirements rose once again and a further chest X-ray showed atelectasis in the right lower and left upper zones. Ventilation was re-started and despite weaning rapidly on the ventilator settings, further attempts at extubation 7 and 11 days later both failed. The Guthrie test was normal.

Questions

1. What is the differential diagnosis?
2. What other investigations are required?

Case 12

A 13-year-old girl had abdominal pain and a fever for 2 days. A pure colony of *Escherichia coli* was grown on urine culture. She was overweight despite having been on several diets, and her weight had markedly increased over the previous 3 months. As a result she was continuously teased at school and was generally rather miserable.

Examination confirmed an unhappy, obese girl (weight 75 kg, height 156 cm), with unsightly acne and a BP of 147/93 mmHg. The neurological examination was normal.

Investigations

Hb, 14.6 g/dl
total white cell count, 16×10^9/l
neutrophils, 12×10^9/l
platelets, 478×10^9/l
Na$^+$, 135 mmol/l
K$^+$, 4.4 mmol/l
urea, 7 mmol/l
urinalysis: more than 1000 white cells per high power field, protein
    3+, red cells 3+, glucose 2+

Questions

1. What further investigations are necessary?
2. What is the diagnosis?

Case 13

A 6-year-old boy developed recurrent flu-like illnesses over a period of 3 months. He presented one month later with a red rash over exposed parts of his body, especially over the face and hands. The problem was not relieved with sunblock creams and 1.0% hydrocortisone cream to the hands. He then developed a painful ulcer over the third knuckle of the right hand. Over this period of time he had become tired and listless, and complained of intermittent pains in his legs. Occasionally he was unable to stand without having to climb up the furniture, and found it difficult to straighten up after bending.

Examination confirmed a thin, withdrawn boy with a facial rash and erythema over the back of the hands and knees. There was moderate lymphadenopathy in the cervical and inguinal groups, and some wasting with diminished power in the quadricep muscles (right worse than left).

Investigations

Hb, 10.2 g/dl
white cell count, $12.4 \times 10^9/l$
lymphocytes, $10.1 \times 10^9/l$
platelets, $631 \times 10^9/l$
ESR, 13 mm in the first hour
ECG, normal
chest X-ray, normal

Questions

1. What investigations are indicated?
2. What is the most likely diagnosis?
3. What treatment is indicated?

Case 14

A 6-month-old girl presented to the local hospital with a fever and cough. She weighed 4 kg. was breathless with marked intercostal recession, a brassy cough, barrel shaped chest cage and inspiratory crepitations.

She was troubled with recurrent possetting and was treated with Gaviscon, thickened feeds and a special homeopathic diet. Two attempts at performing a barium swallow in the prone position had been abandoned as she had become distressed during the procedures. She was a sickly child, and often on antibiotics for respiratory tract infections. She passed 1 – 3 semi-solid stools on alternate days.

14

Investigations

Hb, 8.3 g/dl
total white cell count, 15×10^9/l
neutrophils, 10×10^9/l
lymphocytes, 5×10^9/l
platelets, 223×10^9/l
MCV, 68 fl
blood film, red cells microcytic; hypochromic
faecal occult blood, negative
sweat test, 92 mg of sweat; Na^+ 32 mmol/l; Cl^- 40 mmol/l
chest X-ray, bilateral patchy shadowing in mid-zones and bases

Questions

1. What further investigations are indicated?
2. What is the probable cause for the anaemia?
3. What is the likely diagnosis?

Case 15

A 5-month-old boy presented to casualty with a history of recurrent, uncontrolled seizures over the preceding 12 hours. He had had 3 – 4 loose watery stools for the last 3 days for which no specific treatment was given. He was born normally at term, weighing 3.4 kg. He had been recently vaccinated for the first time though pertussis had been excluded. Vaccination had been delayed as a result of maternal anxiety over the death of a previous son from pneumonia at the age of 3.5 months. Apart from being treated for recurrent thrush, he had been in good health.

On examination he was having generalized clonic seizures. His skin turgor was reduced, the pulse was 102 beats per minute and weak. The BP was 105/65 mmHg and the heart sounds were normal. The respiratory rate was 75 breaths per minute with moderate intercostal recession and bilateral, scattered inspiratory and expiratory crepitations. The anterior fontanelle was tense and muscle tone generally increased. He had profuse, foul smelling semi-solid stools. His condition continued to deteriorate and he lapsed into coma. He died without gaining consciousness after 3 days.

Investigations

Hb, 6.5 g/dl
platelets, 102×10^9/l
total white cell count, 11×10^9/l
neutrophils, 10×10^9/l
Na^+, 126 mmol/l
K^+, 2.6 mmol/l
Ca^{2+}, 2.3 mmol/l
Mg^{2+}, 0.6 mmol/l
glucose, 1.2 mmol/l
chest X-ray, interstitial infiltrate; overexpanded lungs; small heart and narrow mediastinum
urinalysis, no abnormality detected
CSF, white cells 35 per high power field; protein, 2.3 g/l; glucose, 0.5 mmol/l

Questions

1. What should be included in the child's initial management?
2. What investigations are indicated?
3. What led to the child's death?
4. What was the underlying diagnosis?

Case 16

An 8-year-old boy presented to his local hospital with a week's history of intermittent abdominal pain and profuse nocturnal sweating. No abnormality was found on examination and he was allowed home. Four days later, he presented to another hospital with further bouts of severe abdominal pain, not associated with vomiting or any change in bowel habit.

On examination his weight was on the 65th centile, head circumference 95th centile and height on the 60th centile. He was flushed, had several birth marks, skin nodules and slight subcostal tenderness. The temperature was 37.3°C, pulse 110 beats per minute, BP 130/85 mmHg and there was an indistinct fullness in the epigastrium. the symptoms and signs settled and he was sent home, only to return 24 hours later with a similar history as well as diarrhoea. The temperature was 37.2°C, pulse 120 beats per minute and BP 135/85 mmHg. A fullness was palpated in the left upper quadrant but not confirmed on examination 1 hour and again 3 hours later.

Investigations

Hb, 10.2 g/dl
total white cell count, 15×10^9/l
platelets, 200×10^9/l
ESR, 57 mm in the first hour
Na^+, 140 mmol/l
K^+, 3.1 mmol/l
urea, 7 mmol/l
protein, 42 g/l
albumin, 29 g/l

Questions

1. What steps would you have taken on the third admission?
2. What was the cause for the abdominal pain?
3. What was the underlying condition?
4. What complication had arisen?

Case 17

A 10-year-old girl was referred by the school medical officer following a 4 week history of progressive deterioration in speech and gait. Examination revealed a rather shy, pale child who had no skin rashes or signs of jaundice. The pulse was 76 beats per minute, the BP 111/65 mmHg, the heart sounds were normal and the liver edge palpable 2 cm below the costal margin. Though she was able to fully comprehend all that was said to her, she repeated the questions several times over before eventually answering. She demonstrated a fine tremor when asked to show her hands and had a rather curious gait, assuming a hunched posture and walking in short, jerky steps.

Investigations

Hb, 9.4 g/dl
total white cell count, 12.2×10^9/l
platelets, 413×10^9/l
Na^+, 142 mmol/l
K^+, 3.8 mmol/l
urea, 3.6 mmol/l
Ca^{2+}, 2.2 mmol/l
HCO_3^-, 22 mmol/l
total protein, 48 g/l
albumin, 17 g/l
AST, 621 U/l
γGT, 87 U/l
alkaline phosphatase, 311 U/l
urine toxicology, negative
chest X-ray, normal

Questions

1. What is the diagnosis?
2. How can this be confirmed?
3. How would you treat this child?

Case 18

A 14-year-old boy had celebrated his birthday with friends at a local restaurant. On the following day three boys, including the patient, developed acute diarrhoea and abdominal cramps. These symptoms lasted for a period of 2 – 3 days, but all subsequently made a full recovery. Ten days later the patient presented to the local hospital with swelling, pain and limitation of movement in the left ankle and right knee joints. Examination revealed no abnormalities apart from a grossly swollen, tender, warm right knee joint with a grade III effusion, and a red, moderately swollen and tender left ankle. There was marked limitation to full movement in both joints.

Investigations

Hb, 12.3 g/dl
total white cell count, 13.5×10^9/l

neutrophils, $7 \times 10^9/l$
platelets, $421 \times 10^9/l$
ESR 35 mm in the first hour
albumin, 42 g/l
protein, 61 g/l
AST, 50 U/l
ALT, 33 U/l
alkaline phosphatase, 712 U/l
blood cultures, no growth after 48 hours
X-ray right knee, soft tissue swelling of joint; radiolucent area expanding proximal end of fibula with some periosteal reaction
X-ray left ankle, soft tissue swelling of joint

Questions

1. What is the diagnosis?
2. What would be your plan of action?

Case 19

A girl aged 2 years presented with a history of easy bruising and nose bleeds. She weighed 10 kg, measured 65 cm, with a head circumference of 42 cm, had simple low set ears, vestigial thumbs and scattered areas of increased pigmentation over the trunk.

Investigations

Hb, 8.9 g/dl
total white cell count, $3.2 \times 10^9/l$
platelets, $17 \times 10^9/l$
MCV, 97 fl
MCH, 22 pg, MCHC, 29 g/l
HbA, 79%
HbA$_2$, 5%
HbF, 11%
bone marrow aspirate, reduced cellularity with diminished mega-karyocytes

At the age of 4 years she became lethargic and complained of pain in both knees. On examination she was pale and pyrexial.

There was generalized lymphadenopathy and both the liver edge and spleen were palpable 3 cm below the costal margin.

Investigations

Hb, 5.2 g/dl
total white cell count, $21 \times 10^9/l$
neutrophils, $1.8 \times 10^9/l$
platelets, $4 \times 10^9/l$
bone marrow aspirate, markedly hypercellular marrow
X-ray knees, irregular erosions at the metaphyses

Questions

1. What is the underlying diagnosis?
2. How could this diagnosis be confirmed?
3. What change has occurred at the age of four?
4. What is the management for this child?

Case 20

A boy had a history of recurrent bouts of severe abdominal pain and loose, bulky stools. He underwent investigation at the age of 6 years but no underlying cause for his symptoms was discovered. The problem then appeared to have settled and he had enjoyed good health apart from the occasional cold and bout of diarrhoea with mild abdominal pain. At the age of 9 he was admitted to hospital with a severe attack of central abdominal and back pain for 2 days.

He was curled up and disliked being moved or examined. He was in severe distress, sallow, pyrexial, with a pulse of 120 beats per minute, BP of 100/60 mmHg, normal heart sounds, diminished percussion and air entry at the left base. The abdomen was slightly distended, with absent bowel sounds and a firm, tender mass measuring 5×7 cm was palpable in the epigastrium.

Investigations

Hb, 7.3 g/dl
total white cell count, $21 \times 10^9/l$
platelets, $86 \times 10^9/l$
Na^+, 131 mmol/l

K^+, 3.1 mmol/l
HCO_3^-, 17 mmol/l
Ca^{2+}, 2.0 mmol/l
urea, 8.6 mmol/l
creatinine, 0.04 mmol/l
glucose, 14 mmol/l
abdominal X-ray, soft tissue mass with flecks of calcification in the
   upper abdomen

Questions

1. What is the diagnosis?
2. What investigations will help determine the correct diagnosis?
3. How would you manage this patient?

Case 21

A 27-year-old pregnant woman who had registered with this
pregnancy at another hospital, was admitted in labour at 39 weeks'
gestation. She gave birth to a male infant weighing 3.1 kg after a
normal uncomplicated delivery. The baby was well during the first
24 hours but was then noted to become increasingly irritable and
jittery. After a further 12 hours he developed generalized seizures
which did not improve with an intravenous dose of pyridoxine. No
focal neurological deficit could be found on examination, and a
general examination was also normal. At this point the mother
commented that 2 out of 4 previous siblings had had similar
problems after birth.

Investigations

Hb, 10 g/dl
total white cell count, 13×10^9/l
platelets, 128×10^9/l
Na^+, 135 mmol/l
K^+, 3.2 mmol/l
Ca^{2+}, 2.6 mmol/l
PO_4^{3-}, 1.97 mmol/l
Mg^{2+}, 0.78 mmol/l
glucose, 2 mmol/l

serum ammonia, 55 μmol/l
venous pH, 7.22
base deficit, 6
urinalysis, protein 1+
chest X-ray, no abnormality detected
CSF, clear fluid; no cells or organisms seen

Seizure control proved extremely difficult but he was eventually discharged in good health after 5 weeks in hospital.

Questions

1. What further information was required from the presenting history?
2. What treatment was indicated?

Case 22

An infant was born at 37 weeks' gestation to a primigravid mother who tested negative for both rhesus and rubella antibodies. After the initial assessment the mother repeatedly defaulted from the antenatal clinic, and eventually presented in established labour. Delivery was by emergency caesarian section for foetal distress. The Apgar scores were 5 at 1 min and 6 at 5 min. The infant weighed 3.9 kg, measured 50 cm and the head circumference was 35 cm. The baby, umbilical cord and placenta were grossly oedematous, but the skin appeared normal. There was a single umbilical artery but it was impossible to assess for any specific dysmorphic features. The infant was poorly perfused, with a weak pulse of 220 beats per minute, a BP of 43/20 mmHg, and a respiratory rate of 75 breaths per minute with marked subcostal recession. The liver was displaced 3 cm below the costal margin.

Investigations

Hb, 8.3 g/dl
total white cell count, 16×10^9/l
platelets, 122×10^9/l
blood group, O positive

Questions

1. How would you investigate this baby?
2. If the mother had attended the antenatal clinic, what would have been the management?
3. What would be the management after birth?

Case 23

A 3-year-old boy had been investigated for recurrent diarrhoeal episodes. He was found to be on the 60th centile for height and 30th centile for weight. A microcytic anaemia was treated with iron supplements for 4 months.

Two months later, while on holiday visiting friends of the family in another part of the country, he became more miserable and passed between 4–7 offensive, loose stools each day. He was admitted to the nearby childrens' hospital where he was noted to be extremely fractious and was on the 50th centile for height and 3rd centile for weight.

Investigations

Hb, 9.2 g/dl
total white cell count, $13.5 \times 10^9/l$
neutrophils, $6 \times 10^9/l$
lymphocytes, $5 \times 10^9/l$
eosinophils, $1.5 \times 10^9/l$
monocytes, $1 \times 10^9/l$
MCV, 97 fl
MCH, 25 pg
MCHC, 33 g/dl
Na^+, 131 mmol/l
K^+, 3.1 mmol/l
Ca^{2+}, 2.33 mmol/l
urea 7.4 mmol/l
total protein, 62 g/l
albumin, 20 g/l
AST, 32 U/l
IgA, 0.52 g/l

stool, no pathological bacteria grown; *Enterobious vermicularis* ova present
1 hour serum xylose after 5 g oral dose, 0.7 mmol/l
3 day faecal fat, 7.5 g/day

Questions

1. What was the cause of the anaemia at the second presentation?
2. What further investigation is indicated?
3. What is the differential diagnosis?

Case 24

A 13-year-old boy was referred by his GP with a 5 month history of intermittent, severe cramps in both lower limbs, headaches, abdominal pains and 'tingling' in both hands. At times the symptoms appeared to be worse during and after exertion. He was the only child of professional parents, was said to be an academic 'high flier', disliked sports and was rather a loner. He suffered with atopic conjunctivitis, rhinitis and, more recently, a chronic cough.

He was assessed on several occasions by his GP who could not find an abnormality and eventually referred him for a second opinion. He was a well grown, rather anxious boy, with a BP of 140/92 mmHg, prominent conjunctival blood vessels and scattered expiratory wheezes on auscultation. There were two pigmented 'birth marks' on his back, and a few, small, red-blue papules on the medial aspect of both thighs.

Investigations

Na^+, 140 mmol/l
K^+, 4.5 mmol/l
urea, 5 mmol/l
creatinine, 0.05 mmol/l
urinalysis, protein 2+; red cells 1+

Questions

1. What diagnosis best describes this case?
2. What investigations would confirm the diagnosis?

3. What advice should be given to the parents?
4. What pharmacological agent may be of some benefit?

Case 25

A boy aged 14 months had become rather irritable and miserable over the previous 3 weeks and had developed a swelling of the left eye. The 'red eye' reflex on the left was noted to be absent on family photographs take 2 months earlier. Previously he had enjoyed excellent health and had a normal development. He lived with his parents, three older siblings, plus several pets in a large house in the country.

On examination he had shotty lymphadenopathy in the left neck and groins, and the liver edge was palpable 1.5 cm below the costal margin. The right testis was undescended. The left eye was glazed and bulging with a rather indistinct, oedematous appearance compared to the right eye. The red reflex was absent and it was not possible to visualize the retina.

Questions

1. What acute complication has arisen?
2. What is the diagnosis?
3. What steps in the management would you take?

Case 26

A 13-year-old girl presented with a 2 month history of severe headaches not relieved with codeine phosphate. The headaches were particularly severe on waking and during the morning and, as a result, she had been missing school. Her school performance had been deteriorating over a 6 month period, and her parents were concerned that she had dropped out of the top 10 in her class. The symptoms did not appear to be related to her periods which had been regular for the last 6 months. She was a bright child, the youngest of 7 siblings in a close-knit family. The others, aged 21–35 years, were all living away from home. One brother had died suddenly from a subarachnoid haemorrhage the previous year.

She weighed 65 kg, measured 164 cm, and had mild acne, a pulse of 95 beats per minute, BP of 125/70 mmHg, stage III breast and pubic hair development, and a normal neurological examination. She was admitted to hospital where she spent long periods 'moping' in bed, and was noted, intermittently, to have an unsteady gait. After 2 days she complained of additional dizzy spells, weakness and was unable to walk or stand unsupported. On the third night she was found at one end of the ward, lying on the floor, grunting and shaking all four limbs.

Investigations

Na^+, 134 mmol/l
K^+, 4.2 mmol/l
urea, 6 mmol/l
creatinine, 0.03 mmol/l
glucose, 5 mmol/l
ECG, normal
chest and skull X-ray, normal
EEG, no abnormal wave pattern detected during the investigation
CT brain scan with contrast, normal

Question

1. How would you manage this patient?

Case 27

A 10-year-old boy with inflammatory bowel disease and chronic hepatomegaly presented acutely with a temperature of 39.5° C, sweats, rigors and profound lethargy. He had developed mucous diarrhoea 2 days before the admission but had become progressively more drowsy with vomiting and right-sided abdominal pain. His regular medication included alternate day prednisolone, sulphasalazine and overnight nasogastric feeds. As well as recurrent perianal abscesses, he also suffered with skin boils and chest infections.

On examination he appeared flushed, 'clammy', poorly perfused, with a heart rate of 120 beats per minute, BP 105/65 mmHg, and a respiratory rate of 32 breaths per minute. Guarding and tenderness were present over the right upper quadrant. The liver edge was palpable 7 cm below the costal margin. The bowel sounds were reduced and there were old healed scars around the anal verge.

Investigations

Hb, 9.6 g/dl
total white cell count, 14.8×10^9/l
lymphocytes, 12.3×10^9/l
monocytes, 1.2×10^9/l
platelets, 215×10^9/l
ESR, 53 mm in the first hour
Na^+, 132 mmol/l
K^+, 3.2 mmol/l
urea, 7.4 mmol/l
creatinine, 0.07 mmol/l
Ca^{2+}, 2.3 mmol/l
glucose, 1.1 mmol/l
AST, 201 U/l
ALT, 157 U/l
abdominal X-ray, no distended bowel loops; soft tissue shadow in the right upper quadrant

After 6 hours on intravenous fluids, there was an initial improvement and the lethargy and dizziness improved. This was followed by further deterioration with spiking fevers and worsening abdominal pain.

Questions

1. What other investigations are indicated?
2. What has precipitated this admission?
3. What is the underlying condition?

Case 28

An 8-year-old black girl presented to casualty with a 24 hour history of fever and a cough. Examination was unremarkable and the child was allowed to go home. She continued to be unwell and returned to hospital after 48 hours. On examination the temperature was 38.5° C and the tongue was coated. There was slight flaring of the nares, the respiratory rate was 37 breaths per minute, but there were no focal signs on auscultation of the chest. She had just had a chest X-ray in the radiography department when she became stuporose. The emergency team was called. They noted cold peripheries, a pulse of 140 beats per minute and shallow respiratory efforts. The BP was unrecordable. The X-ray was available 7 minutes later and showed consolidation of the right middle lobe. At this point the mother volunteered that her elder son had had a similar problem 2 years previously.

Investigations

Hb, 9.1 g/dl
total white cell count, $27 \times 10^9/l$
neutrophils, $22 \times 10^9/l$
platelets, $312 \times 10^9/l$
blood film, toxic granulation and marked shift to the left
Na^+, 144 mmol/l
K^+, 4 mmol/l
urea, 7.3 mmol/l
pH, 7.22
P_{O_2}, 7.6 kPa
P_{CO_2} 6 kPa
HCO_3^-, 12 mmol/l
base deficit, 8
HIV status, negative

Questions

1. What is the most likely cause for this presentation?
2. How would you manage this child?
3. What further investigations are indicated at a later stage?

Case 29

A 9-week-old baby presented with a 12 hour history of a temp-erature, lethargy, pallor and occasional vomiting of green, discoloured fluid. He seemed to improve on clear fluids, had opened his bowels normally and vomited twice over the next 24 hour period. Twelve hours later the symptoms recurred, and he became rather subdued and irritable when handled. Prior to this episode he had been well since birth, apart from two minor illnesses with vomiting. Examination showed a quiet, listless infant who became markedly frantic when handled. The skin turgor was poor, the pulse 155 beats per minute, BP 55/30 mmHg, respiratory rate 45 breaths per minute, and the bowel sounds were reduced.

Investigations

Na^+, 128 mmol/l
K^+, 2.9 mmol/l
urea, 10.5 mmol/l
creatinine, 0.08 mmol/l
pH, 7.21
HCO_3^-, 12 mmol/l
base deficit, 13

Questions

1. What other investigations may help in this child's management?
2. How would you proceed in the management?
3. What is the diagnosis?

Case 30

A 2½-year-old boy was referred to a paediatric unit following the onset of a progressive blue discoloration of the skin. Though well during infancy, he had become progressively more 'dusky' after the family moved to the country and lived on a farm. He had never been very energetic but there was no recent decrease in his exercise tolerance.

He weighed 15 kg, was not anaemic but had marked central cyanosis in air. The fingers were not clubbed. The BP was 100/65 mmHg, the pulses and the precordium were normal, and there was wide, fixed splitting of the second heart sound. There was a soft 2/6 ejection systolic murmur at the upper left sternal edge. The respiratory rate was 32 breaths per minute, the lung fields were clear and the liver was not palpable below the costal margin.

Investigations

Hb, 11.8 g/dl
total white cell count, $9 \times 10^9/l$
platelets, $322 \times 10^9/l$
ECG, axis 90°; sinus arrhythmia
chest X-ray, normal cardiac size; normal lung fields

Questions

1. What could account for this boy's cardiac signs and general colouring?
2. How would you confirm your suspicions?

Case 31

An 8-year-old girl of West Indian parentage was referred with a 2 month history of intermittent lethargy, aches and pains, 'colds' with nasal catarrh and chest infections. She was rather a thin girl weighing 21 kg, with a temperature of 38°C, a purulent nasal discharge, nasal speech, large tonsils, and inspiratory crepitations at the left base. The liver was palpable 1 cm, and the spleen 3 cm below the costal margins. The symptoms improved in hospital where she received intravenous antibiotics for 7 days, and was allowed home.

Three weeks later she developed a fever, pain in the right thigh and a limp. An X-ray showed no abnormality, but a bone scan showed an area of increased activity in the right femoral shaft. The ESR was 95 mm in the first hour, but several blood cultures were sterile to culture. The symptoms settled after 6 weeks of bed rest and intravenous antibiotics. She was again discharged from hospital but, 2 weeks later, she developed a fever, increasing lethargy, a recurrent nasal discharge and headaches. On examination the weight was 19 kg, the tonsils were enlarged and the spleen was palpable 4 cm below the costal margin.

Investigations

Hb, 8.3 g/dl
total white cell count, 8.8×10^9/l
neutrophils, 6.9×10^9/l
monocytes, 1.2×10^9/l
platelets, 97×10^9/l
absolute reticulocyte count, 0.5%
Coombs' test, negative
Na$^+$, 132 mmol/l
K$^+$, 5.6 mmol/l
urea, 9.7 mmol/l
Ca^{2+}, 2.1 mmol/l
glucose, 6.7 mmol/l
Mantoux and HIV tests, negative
urinalysis, protein 2+; red cells 2+; culture negative
chest X-ray, increased shadowing left base and right mid-zone
abdominal ultrasound, moderate hepatosplenomegaly; no lymph-
    adenopathy
ENT assessment under anaesthesia, increase in soft tissue in nasal
    mucosae, upper airways and Waldeyer's ring

Questions

1. What clinical observations have been omitted?
2. What further investigations are required?
3. What caused the bone lesion?
4. What is the diagnosis?

Case 32

A 14-year-old girl was treated for a cough by her GP For 3 days
before admission to hospital with a 24 hour history of fever and
photophobia. On examination the temperature was 39°C, pulse 130
beats per minute, BP 110/70 mmHg and there was marked nuchal
rigidity. The heart sounds were normal and there was a soft ejection
systolic murmur at the left sternal edge. The breath sounds were
normal.

Investigations

Hb, 10.3 g/dl

total white cell count, 18×10^9/l

Na$^+$, 130 mmol/l

K$^+$, 3 mmol/l

urea, 6.6 mmol/l

glucose, 6 mmol/l

urinalysis, 10 white cells per high power field

CSF, clear; protein 2.2 g/l; glucose 1.2 mmol/l; white cells 55×10^9/l; no organisms were seen on gram stain

She was treated with intravenous cefuroxime for 9 days and was discharged after 10 days. She was perfectly well until she was re-admitted 7 days later with a history of sudden, sharp chest pain followed by a persistent ache and breathlessness. On examination she was clearly in pain. The temperature was 37.4°C, the pulse 155 beats per minute, BP 103/43 mmHg, the chest and heart sounds were normal. A harsh continuous murmur was audible at the base of the heart. The liver was palpable 3.5 cm below the costal margin.

Investigations

Hb, 10 g/dl

total white cell count, 13.8×10^9/l

Na$^+$, 140 mmol/l

K$^+$, 4 mmol/l

glucose, 7 mmol/l

urinalysis, negative

CSF, white cells 5; protein 1.1 g/l; glucose 5 mmol/l; no organisms

chest X-ray, moderate plethora; cardiomegaly

Questions

1. What other investigations are necessary?
2. What steps would be appropriate in the management?
3. What is the diagnosis?

Case 33

A male infant was born at 36 weeks' gestation weighing 2.03 kg, with a head circumference of 31 cm, a diffuse petechial rash, hepatosplenomegaly but normal retinae on fundoscopy. He developed respiratory distress with radiographic evidence of a pneumonitis.

Investigations

Hb, 9.8 g/dl
total white cell count, $7.6 \times 10^9/l$
neutrophils, $0.9 \times 10^9/l$
platelets, $18 \times 10^9/l$
bone marrow aspiration, depleted megakaryocyte numbers
serum bilirubin, 360 μmol/l (direct 207 μmol/l)
ALT, 389 U/l
AST, 903 U/l
alkaline phosphatase, 405 U/l
cranial ultrasound, echogenic enhancement in the caudothalamic grooves and internal capsule
skull X-ray, periventricular calcification
X-rays of the long bones, irregular erosions of the metaphyses
auditory brain-stem evoked responses (BSERs), no response
visual evoked responses (VERs), confirmed cortical visual loss

Questions

1. What is the most likely diagnosis?
2. How would you confirm this?
3. How would you manage this infant?

Case 34

A 12-year-old boy was taken into casualty by his mother. He had developed a swollen, painful left knee, possibly after a fall from his wheelchair. He had had three previous admissions with pneumonia, and required a wheelchair at the age of 10 years following progressive clumsiness and an inability to stand without falling over. Normally a lively, affable boy, he was miserable and withdrawn. He had a temperature of 39° C, a brassy cough, bilateral coarse basal inspiratory crepitations, and a red, warm, swollen, tender left knee joint.

Investigations

Hb, 9.2 g/dl
total white cell count, $8.8 \times 10^9/l$
neutrophils, $7.2 \times 10^9/l$
MCV, 80 fl
MCH, 28 pg
MCHC, 32 g/l
ESR, 56 mm in the first hour
Coombs' test, negative
Na^+, 133 mmol/l
K^+, 3.9 mmol/l
urea, 7 mmol/l
creatinine, 0.04 mmol/l
glucose, 4 mmol/l
IgG, 6.5 g/l
IgM, 0.7 g/l
IgA, 0.01 g/l
IgE, 0.07 g/l
chest X-ray, bilateral streaky shadowing of both bases

Questions

1. How would you investigate this boy?
2. What is the diagnosis?
3. What would constitute the management?

Case 35

A 9-year-old girl was admitted to the local hospital from an institution for physically and mentally handicapped children, where she had been nursed for the past 3 years. She had developed a fever and cough 3 days prior to the admission, then had become drowsy and unresponsive over the preceding 24 hours.

She had been born normally at term to a single, young, unsupported mother. There were early problems with feeding, recurrent 'blue spells' particularly during feeds, and several 'chest infections'. During infancy and early childhood fainting episodes became a common feature of her condition, but these generally

responded to a drink. As a toddler she developed severe behavioural problems which included prolonged head banging and
breath holding attacks. Severe tantrums often resulted in significant
injuries, including fractured bones. Following concern by the social
services, she was transferred to foster parents, but her physical,
behavioural and mental development did not improve. The foster
parents found her behaviour and, in particular, the apparent
disregard for frequent self-injury, impossible to cope with and she
was transferred to the special home.

On admission she was comatose, pyrexial (39.5° C), cyanosed
with diminished breath sounds over the right chest. The right eye
was noted to be red with a shallow corneal abrasion. Both hands and
lips were markedly deformed and showed signs of recent and
previous trauma.

Investigations

Hb, 8.9 g/dl
total white cell count, $25 \times 10^9/l$
neutrophils, $20.6 \times 10^9/l$
platelets, $437 \times 10^9/l$
Na^+, 132 mmol/l
K^+, 4.2 mmol/l
urea, 8.1 mmol/l
urinalysis, protein 1 +

Questions

1. What other investigations are indicated on admission?
2. What would be the initial management?
3. What further investigations would be useful?

Case 36

A 7-year-old girl was being followed up for weight loss in the
general paediatric clinic. The presenting weight was 17 kg and
height 125 cm. The family were known to the local social services as
the father had been imprisoned for illegal possession of cannabis
and heroin. The mother took poor care of herself and suffered with a
chronic, productive cough. The family were notoriously poor clinic

attenders, though whenever seen the child was usually reasonably clean and well dressed.

After a 6 month period of non-attendance the child was brought up to the hospital by a family friend as mother was ill at the time with a chest infection. The child had developed a hacking cough over the preceding 2 months, and had been passing several offensive, loose stools each day for a month. She weighed 15 kg, and an examination revealed multiple verrucae on both hands and reduced air entry at the right base.

Investigations

Hb, 9 g/dl
total white cell count, $13 \times 10^9/l$
neutrophils, $11 \times 10^9/l$
platelets, $111 \times 10^9/l$
Na$^+$, 135 mmol/l
K$^+$, 2.7 mmol/l
urea, 7.5 mmol/l
creatinine, 0.06 mmol/l
albumin, 28 g/l
total protein, 38 g/l
AST, 52 U/l
ALT, 64 U/l
urinalysis, no abnormality detected
chest X-ray, increased shadowing at right base and hilar region

Questions

1. What further investigations are required?
2. What may have caused the diarrhoea?
3. How should this child be managed?

Case 37

A 10-year-old girl was referred to the ENT department with a history of a chronically discharging left ear. The problem had been present, intermittently, for several years and showed a variable response to antibiotics. She was familiar with hospitals and had been under follow-up since the age of 2 years when she had first presented with a limp. An X-ray at that time showed a radiolucent area in the right ilium, just above the acetabulum. At the age of 3 years she had developed pain above the left eye and right shoulder. X-rays showed radiolucent 'punched out' areas in the left superior orbital ridge, right scapula, and cranium. The original lesion in the ilium had disappeared. She then suffered similar problems over the next 7 years, which were managed symptomatically or resolved after short courses of treatment.

She was generally well, though rather small, and had severe seborrhoeic dermatitis of the scalp, deformed nails and crusting with a thick discharge in the left external auditory meatus. It was not possible to view the tympanic membrane on this side.

Investigations

X-rays of the chest, skull, pelvis and limbs, normal
culture left ear, commensals only

Questions

1. What single investigation would be required to confirm the diagnosis?
2. What results would you expect this to show?
3. What is the treatment?
4. What is the prognosis?

Case 38

A 4-year-old girl was brought to casualty with a history of acute malaise, nausea, abdominal pains and headaches. She had been well until 7 days ago when she developed a cold which was treated with paracetamol. Three days prior to this presentation she developed diarrhoea, 6–7 times a day, with foul smelling stools, some of which were blood stained. Despite persisting with oral fluids and 48 hours of ampicillin taken by mouth, her general condition and the diarrhoea continued to deteriorate.

She was miserable, pale with a sallow complexion. The pulse was 125 beats per minute, and a third heart sound was present. There were bilateral basal inspiratory crepitations. The abdomen was distended and diffusely tender with reduced bowel sounds. The liver edge was palpable 2 cm below the costal margin. Shortly after admission she suffered a generalized convulsion.

Investigations

Hb, 5.4 g/dl
total white cell count, 12.3×10^9/l
neutrophils, 10.2×10^9/l
platelets, 59×10^9/l
Na^+, 147 mmol/l
K^+, 6.2 mmol/l
Ca^{2+}, 1.98 mmol/l
HCO_3^-, 13.7 mmol/l
urea, 18 mmol/l
creatinine, 0.32 mmol/l
bilirubin, 27 μmol/l
AST, 170 U/l
chest X-ray, moderate cardiomegaly; bilateral, increased hilar and pulmonary shadowing
abdominal ultrasound, mild hepatomegaly

Questions

1. What caused the generalized convulsion?
2. What further investigations are indicated?
3. What is the management for this child?

Case 39

A 5-year-old boy had been troubled with several flu-like episodes over a 6 month period, with persistent diarrhoea for the last 4 months. He was passing between 3–8 bulky, offensive, semi-solid stools each day and had lost several kilograms in weight. The passage of stool was associated with colicky abdominal pain. Despite the weight loss he was otherwise well and had grown out of two pairs of shoes in the last 3 months. Two years ago he had visited Turkey on holiday with his parents.

Investigations

Hb, 8.8 g/dl
total white cell count, $7.6 \times 10^9/l$
neutrophils, $6.2 \times 10^9/l$
monocytes, $0.7 \times 10^9/l$
platelets, $329 \times 10^9/l$
MCV, 93 fl
MCH, 20 pg
MCHC, 31 g/l
PT, 26 s (control 12 s)
KPPT, 48 s (control 38 s)
TT, 14 s (control 12 s)
corrected times, PT 25 s; KPPT 45 s; TT 12 s
Na^+, 134 mmol/l
K^+, 4.2 mmol/l
Ca^{2+}, 2.1 mmol/l
PO_4^{3-}, 0.6 mmol/l
bilirubin, 8 μmol/l
protein, 33 g/l
alkaline phosphatase, 1032 U/l
AST, 57 U/l
ALT, 69 U/l
abdominal ultrasound scan, no abnormality noted
small bowel meal and follow through, normal
colonoscopy, normal
sweat test, normal
faecal excretion of α_1-antitrypsin, increased

Questions

1. What is the basis for the metabolic problems?
2. What investigations are indicated?
3. What is the underlying abnormality?
4. What treatment is indicated?

Case 40

An 18-month-old boy was brought to casualty by his mother. He had developed a florid rash over both forearms, hands, lower trunk, buttocks and lower limbs over the previous 24 hours. The rash consisted of 0.25 – 0.75 cm circular, in places confluent, erythematous lesions with increased 'redness' in the centre of each lesion with a surrounding 'flare'. A few older lesions on the lower limbs showed signs of bruising. Despite the rash he was relatively well apart from brief episodes when he appeared to be in some distress and drew up his knees as if in pain.

Investigations

Hb, 11.1 g/dl
total white cell count, $8.9 \times 10^9/l$
platelets, $532 \times 10^9/l$
PT, 15 s (control 12 s)
KPPT, 25 s (control 23 s)
TT, 15 s (control 12 s)
INR, 1.1
fibrin degradation products, 13 g/l
urinalysis, red cells 2+; protein 2+
stool, red cells positive; no pathological organisms cultured

Questions

1. What is the diagnosis?
2. How would you manage this child?

Case 41

A 5-year-old girl presented with a 3 day history of abdominal pain. On examination she was frightened and pale. Her respiratory rate was 30 breaths per minute, pulse rate 95 beats per minute, BP 95/60 mmHg and the heart sounds were normal. The abdomen was distended, firm and tender. A large mass was palpable on the right side. Urinalysis showed 2+ blood and 2+ protein. An abdominal ultrasound scan was performed with difficulty as normal structures could not be visualized clearly due to the presence of a large right-sided mass. The aorta was displaced to the left, but the right adrenal gland, right kidney and inferior vena cava could not be identified. Her condition deteriorated over the next 48 hours. On examination at this stage she had a temperature of 37.8° C, a respiratory rate of 40 breaths per minute, a pulse of 120 beats per minute, a BP of 90/55 mmHg, normal heart sounds and a 3/6 pansystolic murmur which was heard best along the left sternal edge.

Questions

1. What is the likely cause for the initial presentation?
2. What complication may have arisen?
3. What investigation was indicated at 48 hours?
4. What would be the management in this situation?

Case 42

A 32-year-old primigravida gave birth to a baby girl weighing 2.9 kg at 37 weeks' gestation. The baby was active but fed poorly from birth. Two hours after the delivery she passed a mucous plug but then did not open her bowels for 3 days. On the evening of the 3rd day she began to vomit frequently. On examination the baby was irritable, the abdomen was distended and the bowel sounds were increased. A plain X-ray of the abdomen showed dilated loops of bowel, and a gastrografin enema showed a small calibre colon containing faecal material. At laparotomy the large bowel was mostly under-developed and there was a particularly narrow segment at the splenic flexure and descending colon. Much of the colon contained meconium. The narrow portion of bowel was resected and a proximal ileostomy and mucous fistula fashioned.

Post-operatively she required assisted ventilation for 3 days on pressures of 30/4, at a rate of 50 breaths per minute and in 45% oxygen. Weaning from the ventilator was delayed by a right mid-zone collapse on the 6th day after birth, and a left upper zone consolidation on the 8th day. She was extubated on the 11th day and nursed in a head box with 60% oxygen. On the 14th day the respiratory rate rose to 65 breaths per minute and she developed marked intercostal and subcostal recession. A chest X-ray showed right mid and lower zone collapse/consolidation and she was re-ventilated. After a further two failed attempts at weaning she was successfully extubated at the age of 26 days, and 3 weeks later was breathing spontaneously in air.

Questions

1. What further investigations are required to make the diagnosis?
2. What steps should be taken in the management of this child?

Case 43

A 10-day-old baby boy presented with a 24 hour history of poor feeding and vomiting. On examination he was poorly perfused with generalized mottling of the skin and required resuscitation with plasma. A beta haemolytic streptococcus was isolated after 2 days incubation in one out of two blood culture bottles taken shortly after admission. He was treated with intravenous amoxycillin and gentamicin for 4 days, made a spectacular recovery and was discharged home on a week's course of amoxycillin given orally.

He was re-admitted 17 days later. Though generally well and active, he had failed to thrive and was refusing to use the left upper limb. The temperature was 37.8° C and he cried each time the left upper arm was handled.

Questions

1. What problem led to the re-admission?
2. How would you criticise the initial management?
3. What further steps are indicated in the management of this child?

Case 44

A 15-year-old Afro-Caribbean boy was brought to casualty by his step father in a semi-comatose state. He had developed a cough 6 days prior to this admission, and was on oral amoxycillin prescribed by his GP. Over the last 36 hours his condition had deteriorated significantly. He had developed frequent vomiting, and became breathless and delirious. At the age of 8 years he was diagnosed and successfully treated for stage IIB Hodgkin's disease involving lymph glands in the neck.

Examination confirmed a well built boy who responded to painful stimuli. He was breathing heavily and had diffuse abdominal tenderness.

Investigations

Hb, 15.5 g/dl
total white cell count, 23×10^9/l
platelets, 392×10^9/l
haematocrit, 58%
ESR, 18 mm in the first hour
Na$^+$, 131 mmol/l
K$^+$, 4.2 mmol/l
urea, 12 mmol/l
serum osmolality, 305 mosmol/l
chest X-ray, overinflated lung fields with streaky shadowing in both bases

Questions

1. What important investigations have been omitted?
2. What is the diagnosis?

Case 45

A neonate was born at 37 weeks' gestation weighing 2.8 kg. Despite an uncomplicated delivery he was distressed at birth with deep cyanosis and marked recession, not relieved by face mask oxygen. An oral endotracheal tube was passed and artificial ventilation commenced. He required a rate of 50 breaths per minute, pressures of 16/2 and 25% oxygen to maintain normal blood gases. Once stabilized, a thorough physical examination showed normal pulses, a normal precordium, normal heart sounds, and a grade 3/6 pansystolic murmur heard all over but best at the lower left sternal edge. There was no hepatomegaly. The left pinna was vestigial with no obvious external auditory canal.

He was extubated at 36 hours of age but became distressed and rapidly developed marked subcostal and suprasternal recession.

Cyanosis, partially improved with crying, was again evident. He was intubated and ventilated on a rate of 40 breaths per minute, pressures of 16/3 and 25% oxygen.

Investigations

glucose, 3.9 mmol/l
blood cultures, negative
CSF, normal
chest X-ray, moderate cardiomegaly and pulmonary plethora
cranial ultrasound, normal

Questions

1. What other clinical examination findings would you require?
2. What investigations would you organize?
3. What is the diagnosis?

Case 46

A 3½-year-old girl was brought to the outpatient department for her 3 monthly assessment for failure to thrive by her foster mother and social worker. She had been born after an uncomplicated pregnancy and delivery. Her mother was an educationally subnormal 35-year-old lady and concerns were voiced early on with regards to her ability to raise a child. At birth the child weighed 2.4 kg, measured 46 cm and had a head circumference of 31 cm. At 12 months of age she weighed 6.1 kg, measured 66 cm and the head circumference was 37 cm. At 18 months she weighed 7.2 kg, measured 71 cm and at this point her name was listed on the 'at risk' register. At the age of 2½ years she weighed 9 kg, measured 77 cm, had a vocabulary of 20 words but was unable to form simple sentences.

She was transferred to foster parents and over the following year she had gained 0.9 kg and had grown 6 cm. She was able to talk in 2–3 word sentences, understood simple commands, copy straight lines and an 'X', and identify 7 animals and name 3 from a picture book. Examination revealed a boisterous, petite girl with rather pixie-like features and particularly small hands.

44

Investigations

glucose, 4.7 mmol/l
thyroxine, 85 nmol/l
growth hormone after provocation test, peak 32 mU/l

Questions

1. What is striking about this child's progress over 3½ years?
2. What may explain the growth pattern?
3. How would you manage this patient?

Weight/height centile charts are available on pages 153 and 154

Case 47

A neonate was born in a district hospital by emergency caesarian section for fetal distress. At birth the Apgar scores were 3 at 1 min and 6 at 5 min and he was noted to have several purple, congested loops of bowel extruding from a defect in the abdominal wall. He was resuscitated with plasma, stabilized on a ventilator, and commenced on antibiotics. The bowel loops were wrapped in warm drapes soaked in betadine before being covered with plastic sheeting. He was transferred to the nearest specialist centre where 15 cm of gangrenous small bowel was resected, an end-to-end anastamosis fashioned and the defect repaired. He made a slow post-operative recovery and remained inactive, unable to tolerate feeds by nasogastric tube and had problems maintaining a normal body temperature. The Guthrie test at 7 days showed a T_4 of 46 nmol/l and TSH of 59 mU/l. A repeat test showed a T_4 of 70 nmol/l and TSH of 121 mU/l. An ultrasound scan of the neck showed a normal thyroid gland. He was commenced on total parenteral nutrition (TPN) and regular T_3 was given intravenously. This was changed to oral T_4 when he began to tolerate nasogastric feeding at the age of 4 weeks. At 6 weeks the T_4 was 105 nmol/l and TSH 4 mU/l, and at 8 weeks the oral T_4 supplements were discontinued. At 10 and 20 weeks the T_4 was 94 nmol/l and 82 nmol/l, and the TSH 1.8 and 2.1 mU/l, respectively.

Investigations

maternal T_4, 110 nmol/l
maternal TSH, 1.7 mU/l
thyroid antibodies (patient), negative
thyroid antibodies (mother), negative
isotope scan at 6 weeks, normal uptake in the thyroid gland

Question

1. What is the explanation for the changes in thyroid function?

Case 48

A 7-year-old girl complained of tingling in her lips on waking in the morning. The problem had occurred intermittently for a period of 2 months and, more recently, had been associated with slurring of her speech and twitching of the right side of the mouth. These symptoms lasted for less than a minute, after which time she would proceed with her usual morning routine. Her GP referred her to the local dentist who diagnosed mild caries of two lower teeth on the right side. Her symptoms persisted and at times she seemed unable to speak prior to leaving for school in the morning. The parents were rather concerned about the possibility of her being bullied at school and had arranged for a meeting with the head teacher. The day before her appointment she developed a 'head cold' and a temperature. That night the parents were woken by a loud cry coming from their daughter's room, and found her to be unresponsive. They noticed that she had right-sided facial twitching which was then followed by generalized shaking of all four limbs for a period of 2 min. The parents rushed her to the nearest hospital, a few minutes drive from their home. On arrival in casualty she was fully conscious but was unable to recall any events since going to bed. An examination, a full blood count, blood chemistry and glucose were found to be normal.

Questions

1. What is the most useful investigation in this case?
2. What would it show?
3. List the main points in the management of this child.

Case 49

A boy had been troubled since the age of 13 months with recurrent bouts of vomiting, abdominal distention and constipation. His growth was poor and he had been fed on several specialized milk feeds to try and improve his weight gain. When he was 2 years old he underwent a series of investigations with the following results:

barium swallow, normal
barium meal and follow through, normal
barium enema, normal
abdominal ultrasound, moderate bilateral megaureters
jejunal biopsy, normal
colonoscopy, normal

He continued to have recurrent bouts of abdominal distension and vomiting, occasionally necessitating admission to hospital. At the age of 4 years he developed profuse vomiting, severe abdominal distension and pain requiring urgent admission to hospital. An examination showed a pale, dehydrated, miserable child with cold peripheries, a pulse of 145 beats per minute, BP of 82/42 mmHg, normal heart sounds, and a uniformly distended abdomen with reduced bowel sounds.

Investigations

Hb, 8.8 g/dl
total white cell count, $18 \times 10^9/l$
platelets, $399 \times 10^9/l$
Na^+, 126 mmol/l
K^+, 2.8 mmol/l
Ca^{2+}, 2.4 mmol/l
HCO_3^-, 17 mmol/l
urea, 17 mmol/l
glucose, 4.3 mmol/l
T_4, 99 mmol/l

TSH, 2.4 mU/l
abdominal X-ray, distended loops of bowel; multiple fluid levels
laparotomy, distended stomach and bowel loops involving the small
    and large bowel; no mechanical obstruction

Questions

1. What immediate steps would you take in managing this child?
2. What investigations may help confirm a diagnosis?
3. What is the diagnosis?

Case 50

A baby girl was born at 37 weeks' gestation to a 22-year-old single
mother. She weighed 2.2 kg, measured 44 cm and had single palmar
creases and epicanthic folds. She developed progressive difficulty
with feeding during the first week of life. The oxygen saturation was
91% in air. Examination showed a gallop rhythm with a grade 2/6
pansystolic murmur at the left sternal edge. The liver was palpable
3 cm below the costal margin. A chest X-ray showed cardiomegaly
and pulmonary plethora and an ECG showed an axis of minus 40°.

She was managed with diuretics and weighed 4.6 kg at the age of
7 months. At this point cardiac catheterization showed a raised
pulmonary arterial pressure which, however, was largely reversible in 100% oxygen. Two months later she went on to have open
heart surgery and a dacron patch was inserted. The post-operative
course was complicated by a central venous line infection and she
was weaned off the ventilator after 15 days. Once on the ward she
continued to feed poorly, failed to gain weight and developed
episodes of generalized mottling and poor perfusion. On examination the temperature was 37.9° C, oxygen saturation 80% in 30%
oxygen, the precordium forceful, and pulse 130 beats per minute.
There was a 3/6 pansystolic murmur at the left sternal edge and
3.5 cm hepatomegaly.

Investigations

Hb, 9.4 g/dl
total white cell count, 14×10^9/l
platelets, 94×10^9/l
Na^+, 136 mmol/l

K^+, 3.4 mmol/l
urea, 8.4 mmol/l
no growth on single blood culture at 48 hours

Her condition continued to deteriorate with increasing breathlessness, pallor and poor perfusion. Continuous oxygen therapy was required in order to maintain an oxygen saturation above 80%. She was re-ventilated and died 12 days later.

Questions

1. What is the underlying heart defect?
2. What investigations were indicated post-operatively?
3. What management was indicated post-operatively?
4. What problem(s) had ultimately led to this child's demise?

Case 51

A boisterous 7-year-old boy was admitted in a state of unconsciousness. He had had a mild upper respiratory infection but had spent the day playing with his older brother in the grounds of the local psychiatric hospital adjacent to their house. The initial examination revealed a temperature of 35.9° C, pulse of 84 beats per minute, BP 95/60 mmHg, normal heart and breath sounds, injected tonsils and a fluid level behind the left tympanic membrane. He was comatose, responding to pain by withdrawal, had slowly reactive pupils, a normal gag reflex, normal fundi and no cranial nerve abnormalities. He was generally hypotonic with diminished deep tendon reflexes though both plantars were flexor. Shortly after admission he suffered two generalized convulsions lasting 3 min each, 30 min apart. A further examination revealed no additional findings.

The parents had recently separated and mother had accused the father of wife battering. The two boys were usually left to play on their own for most of the day and were often in trouble at school for disruptive behaviour.

Investigations

Hb, 11.5 g/dl
total white cell count, 12×10^9/l
neutrophils, 8×10^9/l

platelets, 355×10^9/l
Na^+, 143 mmol/l
K^+, 3.8 mmol/l
Cl^-, 98 mmol/l
Ca^{2+}, 2.3 mmol/l
Mg^{2+}, 0.87 mmol/l
PO_4^{3-}, 1.3 mmol/l
urea, 3.3 mmol/l
creatinine, 0.03 mmol/l
AST, 35 U/l
glucose, 1.3 mmol/l
pH, 7.31
Po_2, 12 kPa
Pco_2, 4.5 kPa
base excess, 3
blood cultures, no growth after 72 hours
chest X-ray, normal
brain CT scan, normal
CSF, normal

Questions

1. How would you manage this child on admission?
2. What other investigation would you request?

Case 52

A girl aged 13 years was involved in a road traffic accident and injured the left knee. On examination in casualty she was pale, quiet and co-operative. She weighed 45 kg, was 132 cm tall with a pulse of 95 beats per minute, a BP of 110/70 mmHg and had no evidence of secondary sexual characteristics. Her left knee joint was swollen, warm and tender with restricted movements.

She was born at term after an uneventful pregnancy, weighed 2.9 kg, measured 45 cm and had a head circumference of 31 cm. Her mother admitted that, as an active toddler, she had sustained several injuries and was forever covered in bruises compared with her siblings. At 4 years of age she had tripped on the carpet and had developed a swollen, tender left elbow joint, for which she was admitted to hospital for 48 hours. Records at the time showed that she weighed 14 kg, measured 88 cm and her development was appropriate for her age.

Investigations

Hb, 9.7 g/dl
total white cell count, 7.9 × 10⁹/l
platelets, 320 × 10⁹/l
PT, 13 s (control 12 s)
KPPT, 41 s (control 26 s)
TT, 12 s (control 10 s)
factor VIII, 5% of the normal amount
von Willebrand factor, normal

Questions

1. What is the reason for the swollen knee?
2. How could this condition be explained in this particular girl?

Weight/height centile charts are available on pages 153 and 154

Case 53

A 6-year-old girl was referred to a paediatric gastroenterology centre for the investigation of persistent vomiting. She had been a bright and healthy girl. Shortly after the family returned to the UK from South-East Asia, she developed intermittent bouts of vomiting. These were initially sporadic, but over the next 4 weeks had increased in frequency. Vomiting usually occurred shortly before breakfast. Occasionally she would vomit up to 6–7 times a day, complain of headaches and then refuse to go to school. At times the vomitus would become bile stained and streaked with blood. Her appetite had deteriorated considerably and she had lost 1.6 kg in weight.

Investigations

Hb, 8.3 g/dl
total white cell count, 15 × 10⁹/l
platelets, 236 × 10⁹/l
MCH, 22 pg

MCHC, 30 g/dl
Na^+, 141 mmol/l
K^+, 3.3 mmol/l
Cl^-, 110 mmol/l
HCO_3^-, 25 mmol/l
urea, 5.8 mmol/l
creatinine, 0.1 mmol/l
glucose, 6.2 mmol/l
barium swallow, normal

A gastroscopy was organized. The day before the gastroscopy she vomited twice and was drowsy and subdued all day long.

Questions

1. What clinical assessment was indicated prior to the gastroscopy?
2. What investigation is indicated?

Case 54

A 6-year-old boy was on maintenance treatment for acute lympho-blastic leukaemia (ALL). He had received a dose of intravenous vincristine and a 5 day course of oral prednisolone at the start of the month in accordance with the standard protocol for ALL. When reviewed 14 days later, his mother commented that he had been unwell over the preceding 24 hours. He had been complaining of abdominal pain and had vomited four times. The pain was not relieved after a normal bowel action that same morning, and persisted so that he had to be carried into the clinic. Nevertheless, he managed to lift himself onto the couch. There was minimal periumbilical abdominal tenderness, but no other abnormality on examination and he was sent home with mild analgesic medication.

He was re-admitted the following day with similar symptoms. On examination he looked unwell and was febrile (38° C), with a pulse of 110 beats per minute, a BP 95/55 mmHg and a respiratory rate of 40 breaths per minute. There was diffuse periumbilical and right sided abdominal pain with mild guarding but no rebound tender-ness. He seemed most comfortable when placed prone with the right lower limb flexed at the hip.

Question

1. What is the diagnosis?

Case 55

A 19-month-old South Asian boy was brought to casualty by his mother who was concerned that he seemed unable to walk. The problem appeared to have deteriorated during a recent illness with diarrhoea and vomiting. He was born at term, weighing 3.1 kg and had fed well. He sat unsupported at the age of 7 months, had rolled from the supine to the prone position aged 9 months, and cruised around the furniture at 12 months. At the age of 14 months he was able to walk with one hand held, but he had refused to weight bear on the lower limbs over the past 2 months.

Examination revealed a miserable, pale, slightly dehydrated child. The liver edge was palpable 1.5 cm below the costal margin, and both wrists and knees appeared to be swollen. There was no obvious area of tenderness over the back and lower limbs, though the power in the limbs was generally reduced and he was unable to stand.

Investigations

Hb, 8.4 g/dl
total white cell count, 13.6×10^9/l
platelets, 322×10^9/l
blood film, red cells microcytic; hypochromic
Na^+, 133 mmol/l
K^+, 3.4 mmol/l
Cl^-, 98 mmol/l
Ca^{2+}, 2.1 mmol/l
Mg^{2+}, 0.8 mmol/l
PO_4^{3-}, 0.6 mmol/l
HCO_3^-, 23 mmol/l
urea, 7.3 mmol/l
creatinine, 0.06 mmol/l
bilirubin, 9 μmol/l
AST, 49 U/l
ALT, 60 U/l

Questions

1. What other information would you require from the history?
2. What other investigative results would you require?
3. What is the most probable diagnosis?

Case 56

A 9-year-old-boy was referred from abroad for further investigation. He had developed progressive abdominal distention over a period of 7 months, and had reduced exercise tolerance compared to his peers.

Examination revealed a frightened but co-operative child who did not speak any English. He was pale, anicteric and weighed 38 kg. Congestion of the jugular veins was evident on deep inspiration. The pulse varied between 90–97 beats per minute and the heart sounds were normal. Auscultation of the chest revealed a few coarse crackles in the bases. The abdomen was uniformly distended and a firm liver edge was palpable 10 cm below the costal margin. The spleen measured 2 cm below the costal margin. Shifting dullness was easy to elicit and there was pitting oedema above both ankles.

Investigations

Hb, 10.1 g/dl
total white cell count, $14.4 \times 10^9/l$
platelets, $238 \times 10^9/l$
Na^+, 139 mmol/l
K^+, 4.5 mmol/l
urea, 6.4 mmol/l
HCO_3^-, 19 mmol/l
bilirubin, 22 μmol/l
total protein, 48 g/dl
albumin, 24 g/dl
AST, 73 U/l
ALT, 98 U/l
γGT, 64 U/l

chest X-ray; normal sized heart; flecks of calcification at the right
hilum; prominent vascular markings with Kerley B lines at both
bases
abdominal ultrasound, uniform hepatosplenomegaly; ascites

Questions

1. What other physical sign would be useful in the clinical assessment of this case?
2. What further investigations are required?
3. What is the diagnosis?
4. What is the treatment?

Case 57

After an uneventful pregnancy, a 26-year-old woman gave birth at
term to an apparently healthy baby girl who weighed 3.1 kg. She
was active, fed well and gained weight but was referred to the
hospital at 12 days of age. The midwife had noted progressive,
generalized yellow discoloration of the skin and pale stools. On
examination the liver edge was palpable 1.5 cm below the costal
margin. The splenic tip was also palpable.

Investigations

Hb, 13 g/dl
total white cell count, $18 \times 10^9/l$
neutrophils, $11 \times 10^9/l$
platelets, $432 \times 10^9/l$
Na^+, 137 mmol/l
K^+, 3.8 mmol/l
urea, 5.7 mmol/l
creatinine, 0.04 mmol/l
Ca^{2+}, 2.7 mmol/l
bilirubin, 127 μmol/l
albumin, 38 g/l
alkaline phosphatase, 440 U/l
AST, 104 U/l
γGT, 241 U/l
urine and serum amino acids, normal

urinalysis, sterile; no reducing substances
ultrasound scan, normal liver parenchyma and gall bladder
immunoreactive trypsin (IRT), normal
hepatobiliary scintigraphy, impaired uptake in liver and slow
  excretion into duodenum

Questions

1. What further investigations are indicated?
2. What is the most probable diagnosis?
3. What is the management?

Case 58

A girl of Middle-Eastern origin had been followed up for failure to thrive. She had weighed 3.0 kg at birth but despite a good appetite, had grown poorly. She had always been the shortest in her class but made up for her lack of height with a sharp mind and good sense of humour. Her parents were 4th cousins and she had three brothers whose height plotted on the 10th centile.

When first measured, aged 7 years, the height was 92 cm and weight 16.5 kg. She was commenced on a trial of growth hormone, and received 0.1 units/m^2/day by subcutaneous injection on 4 days per week, for a period of 2 years. At the age of 9 years the height was 100.5 cm and weight 19 kg. Therapy was continued for another 36 months with a poor response, and she was then referred for a second opinion.

Examination showed a well-adjusted, bright young lady who measured 115 cm and weighed 26 kg. The visual fields were normal. Secondary sexual characteristics included stage II breast and pubic hair development but, on direct questioning, she had yet to commence menses. Her intellectual skills were assessed to be appropriate for a girl of her age.

Investigations

Na$^+$, 140 mmol/l
K$^+$, 4.3 mmol/l
urea, 2.8 mmol/l
creatinine, 0.04 mmol/l
T$_4$, 87 nmol/l

TSH, 2.1 mU/l
bone age, consistent with a girl aged 10.5 years
0900 hrs cortisol, 504 mmol/l
2400 hrs cortisol, 258 mmol/l
peak growth hormone after insulin provocation test, 122 mU/l

Questions

1. What is the diagnosis?
2. What treatment may be employed?

Weight/height charts are available on pages 153 and 154

Case 59

A 3-year-old girl was referred by her GP who was concerned by the recent appearance of multiple bruises over her body. The mother was herself rather concerned about her child's bruising which she had noticed over the preceding 24 hours. She admitted that her daughter was rather lively and was never free of bruises over the knees and shins. She could account for some of the new bruises as her daughter had fallen over and grazed the right shin the previous morning and, later in the day, had crashed into a door at home, hitting her forehead. However, the subsequent bruises appeared to be much darker than usual. Apart from a cold 5 days before, she had been in good health.

On further questioning mother admitted that she was a reformed heroin addict. She had become involved in an intensive programme run by the local drug addiction unit and had discontinued methadone 6 months before this referral. She was currently maintained on a reducing dose of diazepam and amitryptyline, 50 mg once every night.

Though initially apprehensive, the child soon adjusted to the strange environment and a thorough examination was possible. The temperature was 37° C, there were no signs of anaemia or generalized lymphadenopathy. There was a haematoma on the upper lip and slight bleeding from the gingival margins. Her body was covered in multiple bruises varying in size and colour. There was a fresh graze over the right shin with marked bruising, and a haematoma over the left side of the forehead as well as over the right flank and left knee. There was a superficial, macular, non-blanching erythematous rash over the eyelids, cheeks, earlobes, neck, chest, abdominal wall and left groin.

Questions

1. What single investigation is indicated?
2. What is the most likely diagnosis?

Case 60

A 10-year-old boy presented with a generalized convulsion lasting 20 min. He had had a mild upper respiratory tract infection and was found to have a temperature of 37.8° C for 24 hours prior to the convulsion, but had been well apart from occasional 'tension' headaches since changing schools 6 months ago.

His pulse was 125 beats per minute, BP 174/96 mmHg (right arm) and 164/92 mmHg (right leg), the apex beat was forceful in nature and there was a grade 1/6 ejection systolic murmur at the base of the heart and a grade 3/6 systolic murmur over the back and abdomen. Neurological assessment, including fundoscopy, was normal. A cranial CT scan was reported to be normal. He had two further generalized seizures over the next 24 hours.

Questions

1. What therapeutic measures are indicated?
2. What investigations are indicated?
3. What is the diagnosis?

Answers and discussions

Case 1

Answers

		Score
1.	Abdominal ultrasound or abdominal CT (+3), biopsy mass (+3).	(+6)
2.	Beckwith–Wiedemann syndrome (or exomphalos-macroglossia-gigantism (EMG) syndrome).	(+4)
		(+10)

Others

Q1: α feto-protein (+1), human chorionic gonadotrophin (HCG) (+1), chest X-ray (+1); CT chest (+0.5), bone scan (+0.5), bone marrow (+0.5).

Q2: Infant of diabetic mother (+2).

(Average)

Discussion

The diagnosis of Beckwith–Wiedemann syndrome should be considered in view of the gigantism and transient asymptomatic hypoglycaemia in the neonatal period. These children often have visceromegaly that cannot be contained within the neonatal abdominal wall and present with an exomphalos. In this infant incomplete closure of the abdominal wall had resulted in a large umbilical hernia. Other associations of this syndrome include hemihypertrophy, transverse creases on the earlobes, skin haemangiomas and an increased risk for developing malignant disease. At 10 months of age any abdominal mass should be presumed to be malignant, and the differential diagnosis of a right-sided abdominal mass should include nephroblastoma, hepatoblastoma and neuroblastoma. Both the first two are associated with the Beckwith–Wiedemann syndrome, though the thrombocytosis seen on the peripheral blood count is more suggestive of hepatoblastoma. The dilemma is best resolved by good imaging techniques (i.e. ultrasound which is easily available and inexpensive, or CT scanning), and histological examination of a biopsy specimen. Other investigations are important in staging procedures, and, like the presence of tumour markers, may be highly suggestive though not diagnostic for the condition.

Further reading

Beckwith–Wiedemann syndrome. In *Nelson Textbook of Pediatrics*, 14th edn, Behrmann R.E. (ed). W.B. Saunders, Philadelphia, pp. 413 (1992)

Beckwith–Wiedemann syndrome. In *Forfar and Arneil's Textbook of Paediatrics*, 4th edn, Campbell A.G.M., McIntosh N. (eds). Churchill Livingstone, London, pp. 323 (1992)

Hepatoblastoma and Beckwith–Wiedemann syndrome. In *Forfar and Arneil's Textbook of Paediatrics*, 4th edn, Campbell A.G.M., McIntosh N. (eds). Churchill Livingstone, London, pp. 1000 (1992)

Beckwith–Wiedemann syndrome. In *Smith's Recognizable Patterns of Human Malformation*, 4th edn, Jones K.L. (ed). W.B. Saunders, Philadelphia, pp. 136–139 (1988)

WEINBERG A.G., FINEGOLD M.J. Primary hepatic tumours in childhood. In *Pathology of Neoplasia in Children and Adolescents*, Finegold M.J. (ed). W.B. Saunders, Philadelphia, pp. 333–372 (1986)

Case 2

Answers

		Score
1.	Munchausen syndrome by proxy.	(+4)
2.	Urine and serum osmolality profiles off DDAVP with mother absent.	(+6)
		(+10)

(Easy)

Discussion

The diagnosis of diabetes insipidus is immediately brought into question when the patient was found to be able to concentrate the urine above 200 mosmol/l without the need of DDAVP. The realization that the normal physiological process could proceed with the mother inadvertently absent, suggests that the mother was in some way responsible for the abnormal results. Indeed, she had been systematically diluting the child's urine with tap water! Confirmation of the diagnosis would involve a clear, repeatable demonstration of the normal urinary concentrating powers in this patient, without any interference or supervision from mother and, if necessary, under the protection of a suitable court order.

Further reading

Munchausen by proxy. In *Nelson Textbook of Pediatrics*. 14th edn, Behrman R.E. (ed). W.B. Saunders, Philadelphia, pp. 972 (1992)

MEADOW R. Munchausen syndrome by proxy. *Archives of Disease in Childhood*, **57**, 92–98 (1982)

MEADOW R. Management of Munchausen syndrome by proxy. *Archives of Disease in Childhood*, **60**, 385–393 (1985)

Case 3

Answers

		Scores
1.	Kawasaki disease.	(+1)
2.	Anti nuclear cytoplasmic antibodies (ANCA) (+0.5), ECG (+0.5), echocardiogram (+0.5), antistreptococcal titres (ASOT) (+0.5), platelet count (+0.5), white cell count (+0.5).	(+3)
3.	Myocardial ischaemia due to coronary aneurysm(s).	(+1)
4.	Repeat echocardiogram (+0.5), cardiac enzymes and serial ECGs (+0.5).	(+1)
5.	Aspirin (+1), immunoglobulin (+1), treat heart failure (+1); dipyridamole (+0.5), prostacyclin (+0.5).	(+3) (+1)
		(+10)

62

Others

Q2: Blood culture (+0.25), viral titres (+0.25), clotting profile (+0.25), immunoglobulins (+0.25), complement C_3, C_4 (+0.25).

(Easy)

Discussion

The combination of symptoms and signs presented in this case make Kawasaki syndrome the most likely diagnosis. Indeed, this diagnosis is based on clinical criteria, namely:
- Persistent fever for at least 5 days.
- Any 4 of the following:
  cervical lymphadenopathy
  polymorphous skin rash
  mucositis, strawberry tongue
  bilateral, non-purulent conjunctivitis
  peripheral oedema, skin desquamation
- Illness not explained by other disease processes.

Other symptoms and complications may include a cough, abdominal pain, diarrhoea, vomiting, transient arthralgia, aseptic meningitis, nerve palsies, sterile pyuria and gall bladder hydrops. The most serious complication involves a vasculitic process affecting major arteries including the coronaries. Coronary aneurysms may occur in 10–40% of patients within the first 2 weeks of the illness. Thrombosis and frank myocardial infarction may develop, as well as cardiac failure, myocarditis, pericarditis, arrhythmias and rarely aneurysmal rupture. A leucocytosis is common in the first week and a thrombocytosis during the second and third week. The ESR, C-reactive protein, ANCA and complement levels are usually raised. Treatment includes: gamma immunoglobulin as a single dose of 2 g/kg, which, if given in the acute phase, may reduce the degree of cardiac damage; aspirin, 100 mg/kg/day in divided doses for 2 weeks and 3–5 mg/kg/day for 6–8 weeks (or until coronary aneurysms resolve). Anticoagulants (heparin or warfarin), thrombolytic agents (streptokinase) and prostacyclin are indicated in patients with proven coronary artery thrombosis.

Further reading

Kawasaki disease. In *Nelson Textbook of Pediatrics*, 14th edn, Behrmann R.E. (ed). W.B. Saunders, Philadelphia, pp. 627–631 (1992)

Kawasaki disease. In *Forfar and Arneil's Textbook of Paediatrics*, 4th edn, Campbell A.G.M., McIntosh N. (eds). Churchill Livingstone, London, pp. 1536–1538 (1992)

KAWASAKI T., KOSAKI F., OKAWA S., SHIGEMATSU I. and YANAGAWA H. A new infantile acute febrile mucocutaneous lymph node syndrome (MLNS) prevailing in Japan. *Pediatrics*, **54**, 271–276 (1974)

SHULMAN S.D., BASS J.L., BIERMAN F., *et al*. Management of Kawasaki syndrome: A consensus statement prepared by North American participants of the Third International Kawasaki Disease Symposium, Tokyo, Japan. December 1988. *Pediatric Infectious Disease Journal*, **8**, 663–665 (1989)

SAVAGE C.O.S., TIZARD J., JAYNE D., LOCKWOOD C.M. and DILLON M.J. Antineutrophil cytoplasm antibodies in Kawasaki disease. *Archives of Disease in Childhood*, **64**, 360–363 (1989)

Case 4

Answers

		Scores
1.	Stool culture (+1); blood or bone marrow cultures (+1); blood film for parasites (+1).	(+3)
2.	*Salmonella typhi* infection (+1.5), malaria (+1.5).	(+3)
3.	Antibiotics: cefuroxime, chloramphenicol or ciprofloxacin (+1), antipyretics (+1); antimalarials (+1); isolation (+1).	(+4)
		(+10)

Others

Q2: Enterobacter infection (+0.5).

(Average)

Discussion

This child presented with symptoms consistent with an infection probably acquired outside the UK. Salmonellosis and malaria must be considered. In view of the abdominal (rose) spots, salmonellosis is the more likely diagnosis. Multi-resistant organisms (especially to ampicillin and chloramphenicol) are becoming more common worldwide, and treatment with cefuroxime or ciprofloxacin may be necessary. *Salmonella typhi* antigen serology is usually positive in the second week of the illness, though the organism may be grown in blood and stool cultures within 7 days. In partially treated cases, culture of a bone marrow aspirate may provide the answer. In this case malaria will need to be excluded by inspection of a thick blood film for parasites. Apart from the use of specific anti-microbial agents, the management should include temperature control and nursing in isolation.

Further reading

Malaria. In *Nelson Textbook of Pediatrics*, 14th edn, Behrmann R.E. (ed). W.B. Saunders, Philadelphia, pp. 876–879 (1992)

Malaria. In *Forfar and Arneil's Textbook of Paediatrics*, 4th edn, Campbell A.G.M., McIntosh N. (eds). Churchill Livingstone, London, pp. 1503–1510 (1992)

Salmonella typhi. In *Nelson Textbook of Pediatrics*, 14th edn, Behrmann R.E. (ed). W.B. Saunders, Philadelphia, pp. 730–731 (1992)

Salmonella typhi. In *Forfar and Arneil's Textbook of Paediatrics*, 4th edn, Campbell A.G.M., McIntosh N. (eds). Churchill Livingstone, London, pp. 1380 (1992)

VALLENAS C., HERNANDEZ H., BRADLEY, K., BLACK R. and GOTUZZO E. Efficacy of bone marrow, blood, stool and duodenal contents culture for bacteriological confirmation of typhoid fever in children. *Pediatric Infectious Disease Journal*, **4**, 486–498 (1985)

WICKS A.C.B., HOMES G.S. and DAVIDSON L. Endemic typhoid fever. *Quarterly Journal of Medicine*, **159**, 341–354 (1971)

Case 5

Answers

		Scores
1.	Hereditary spherocytosis or congenital haemolytic anaemia.	(+2)
2.	Osmotic fragility tests (+2), autohaemolysis tests (+2), viral serology (+2).	(+6)
3.	Hypoplastic crisis secondary to parvovirus.	(+2)
		(+10)

Others

Q1: Leukaemia (+1).

Q2: Bone marrow aspiration (+1), haemoglobin electrophoresis (+1).

(Hard)

Discussion

This child was anaemic and icteric. The raised bilirubin level was predominantly unconjugated and therefore probably the result of haemolysis. The peripheral blood picture showed a pancytopenia, the reticulocyte count was low (in the presence of haemolysis) and the Coombs' test was negative, suggesting marrow hypofunction. A haemolytic anaemia in crisis was therefore a distinct possibility. Hereditary spherocytosis and β-thalassaemia should be considered since the spleen was palpable and the red cells were microcytic. It would be unusual for children with sickle cell disease to have a palpable spleen at this age. Infections due to mycoplasma and infectious mononucleosis may be associated with a similar clinical scenario, but the haemolytic anaemia in these instances is the result of an autoimmune process and would be Coombs' positive. Acute leukaemia presenting with pancytopenia was a possible diagnosis but would not explain the unconjugated hyperbilirubinaemia. Children with congenital haemolytic anaemia may develop an acute haemolytic crisis or an aplastic/hypoplastic crisis, often following an infection with parvovirus. During an aplastic crisis severe anaemia is accompanied by leucopenia and thrombocytopenia, though the serum bilirubin level may remain only moderately elevated. Hereditary spherocytosis is inherited in an autosomal dominant fashion – indeed, this boy's sister presented with identical symptoms and signs 7 days later!

Further reading

Hereditary spherocytosis. In *Nelson Textbook of Pediatrics*, 14th edn, Behrmann R.E. (ed). W.B. Saunders, Philadelphia, pp. 1242–1243 (1992)

Hereditary spherocytosis. In *Forfar and Arneil's Textbook of Paediatrics*, 4th edn, Campbell A.G.M., McIntosh N. (eds). Churchill Livingstone, London, pp. 928–929 (1992)

KELLEHER J.H., LUBAN N.L.C., MORTIMER P.P. and KAMIMURA T. Human serum parvovirus: A specific cause of aplastic crisis in children with hereditary spherocytosis. *Journal of Pediatrics*, **102**, 720–722 (1983)

EBER S.W., ARMBRUST R. and SCHROTER W. Variable clinical severity of hereditary spherocytosis. Relation to erythrocytic spectrum concentration, osmotic fragility and autohaemolysis. *Journal of Pediatrics*, **117**, 409–416 (1990)

Case 6

Answers

Scores

1. Blood gas in 100% oxygen (+1), echocardiogram
   (+1), blood cultures (+1).   (+3)
2. Antibiotics (+1), prostaglandin E (+1), ventilation
   (+1), correct acidosis (+1), dextrose (+1).   (+5)
3. Obstructed (infradiaphragmatic) total anomalous
   pulmonary venous drainage.   (+2)

(+10)

(Average)

Discussion

This neonate presented with poor perfusion and marked breath-lessness at the age of 7 days. Since the examination on day 5 was normal, the subsequent deterioration could be explained by closure of the ductus arteriosus in a duct-dependent congenital heart disease (CHD). The most likely lesions to present at this age would include transposition of the great arteries (TGA), pulmonary (PA) and tricuspid atresia (TA), hypoplastic left heart (hypo LH) and total anomalous pulmonary venous drainage (TAPVD). As shown in the table below, obstructed TAPVD (obs) would best explain the investigative results presented in this case.

In TAPVD the four pulmonary arteries do not connect with the left atrium. Instead they connect with the right atrium, directly or via large veins in the mediastinum (and produce the classical figure-of-eight/snowman/cottage loaf appearance on the chest X-ray). Alternatively they join into a confluence of veins that empties via a long descending vein into the portal or hepatic venous systems. Venous obstruction at these sites is common – obstruction at the level of the hepatic veins may result in large venous lakes with the liver. The subsequent poor venous return results in underfilling of the heart (and therefore no cardiomegaly on chest X-ray), and severe pulmonary venous congestion with right ventricular hyper-trophy.

Cyanotic CHD presenting within 4 weeks: ECG and chest X-ray results

Lesion	ECG	Chest X-ray
TGA	Normal R dominance	Mild cardiomegaly; plethora
TGA (+VSD)	R or R+L hypertrophy	Cardiomegaly; plethora
TGA(+VSD+PS)	RAD; R+L hypertrophy	Cardiomegaly; normal lung fields
TAPVD	RV hypertrophy	Cardiomegaly (unobstructed) No cardiomegaly (obstructed) Pulmonary plethora
Hypo LH	RV hypertrophy	Cardiomegaly; plethora
PA (no VSD)	RAD + mild RV hypertrophy	Pulmonary oligaemia
PA (+VSD)	RAD; RV hypertrophy	Pulmonary oligaemia
TA	Superior axis/LAD	Pulmonary oligaemia

R = right; L = left; RAD = right axis deviation; LAD = left axis deviation; RV = right ventricle; LV = left ventricle; VSD = ventricular septal defect; PS = pulmonary stenosis.

Further reading

Total anomalous pulmonary venous return. In *Nelson Textbook of Pediatrics*, 14th edn, Behrmann R.E. (ed). W.B. Saunders, Philadelphia, pp. 1159–1160 (1992)

Total anomalous pulmonary venous return. In *Forfar and Arneil's Textbook of Paediatrics*, 4th edn, Campbell A.G.M., McIntosh N. (eds). Churchill Livingstone, London, pp. 694–695 (1992)

CLARKE D.R., STARK J., DE LEVAL M., PINCOTT J.R. and TAYLOR J.F.N. Total anomalous pulmonary venous return in infancy. *British Haematology Journal,* **39,** 436–444 (1977)

TURLEY K., TUCKER W.Y., ULLYOT D.J. and EBERT P.A. Total anomalous pulmonary venous connection in infancy. Influence of age and type of lesion. *American Journal of Cardiology,* **45,** 92–97 (1980)

Case 7

Answers

Scores

1. Intravenous dextrose (+1), increase ventilation
   pressure (+1), septic screen followed by
   antibiotics (+1).   (+3)
2. Ultrasound abdomen (+1), urinary electrolytes
   (+0.5), repeat septic screen (+0.5).   (+2)
3. Dextrose (+1), blood transfusion (+1), intravenous
   hydrocortisone and fludrocortisone (+1).   (+3)
4. Adrenal haemorrhage.   (+2)

(+10)

Others

Q3: Lower serum potassium (+0.5), give calcium (+0.5).

(Hard)

Discussion

This question centres around the differential diagnosis of the causes of a collapse in an artificially ventilated neonate. This infant had a poor Apgar score at birth with a severe respiratory acidosis and evidence of hyaline membrane disease on the chest X-ray. She had been making steady progress at the time of the collapse, 83 hours after birth. The predominantly metabolic rather than respiratory acidosis would argue against a pneumothorax. However, the clotting profile was abnormal and the haemoglobin had fallen by 4.5 g/dl, suggestive of a recent haemorrhage. An intraventricular bleed seemed unlikely in view of the result of the cranial ultrasound. However, the presence of persistent hypotension, hypoglycaemia, hyponatraemia and hyperkalaemia would suggest adrenal dysfunction secondary to an adrenal haemorrhage. The latter may be evident as a palpable abdominal mass and should be seen on abdominal ultrasound scanning. As sepsis cannot be ruled out as a cause for this baby's collapse and metabolic derangements, the management would require screening for infection and antibiotic cover, as well as correction of the anaemia and metabolic abnormalities.

Further reading

Haemorrhage into the adrenal gland. In *Nelson Textbook of Pediatrics*, 14th edn, Behrmann R.E. (ed). W.B. Saunders, Philadelphia, pp. 457, 1443 (1992)

Adrenal haemorrhage. In *Forfar and Arneil's Textbook of Paediatrics*, 4th edn, Campbell A.G.M., McIntosh N. (eds). Churchill Livingstone, London, pp. 1140 (1992)

HILL E.E. and WILLIAMS J.A. Massive adrenal haemorrhage in the newborn. *Archives of Disease in Childhood*, **34**, 178–182 (1959)

Case 8

Answers

		Score
1.	Ultrasound renal tracts (+2), urine for culture and microscopy (+2), calcium/creatinine ratio (+2);	(+6)
	abdominal X-ray (+1), 24 hour oxalate excretion (+1), intravenous urogram (+1), micturation cysto-urethrogram (+1).	(+4)
		(+10)
		(Easy)

Discussion

The combination of renal colic and haematuria suggested renal calculi as a possible diagnosis. Renal stones are rather less common in western countries than in other parts of the world. They may be radio-opaque (calcium infection-related stones), slightly radio-opaque (cystine stones), or radioluscent but detectable on ultrasound imaging (uric acid, xanthine stones). The investigation for renal calculi should exclude: urinary tract infection, urinary stasis, obstruction and reflux. Crystallography on the urine may reveal the nature of the calculi. Metabolic analysis should include: the estimation of the serum calcium, phosphate, uric acid and creatinine levels; urine pH, calcium:creatinine ratio and creatinine clearance; 24 hour urinary excretion of calcium, phosphate, oxalate, uric acid and amino acids. Idiopathic isolated hypercalciuria without hypercalcaemia resulting in calcium oxalate stones is often the diagnosis. However, hypercalcaemia will require further investigation to exclude conditions such as hyperthyroidism, hypervitaminosis D and sarcoidosis. Stone formation is also a feature in patients with renal tubular acidosis, cystinuria, xanthinuria, hyperoxaluria, hyperuricaemia and nephrocalcinosis. Infections, particularly with Proteus species, can result in the precipitation of magnesium/ammonium/phosphate and calcium phosphate stones. The treatment involves surgery or lithotripsy for unusually large stones and those associated with obstruction. Adequate hydration and maintenance of a diuresis is essential, and any urinary infection must be eradicated. Alkalinization of the urine is beneficial with cystine and uric acid stones, and allopurinol is the drug of choice for uric acid and xanthine stones.

Further reading

Calculi and haematuria. In *Nelson Textbook of Pediatrics*, 14th edn, Behrmann R.E. (ed). W.B. Saunders, Philadelphia, pp. 1380 (1992)

Renal stones. In *Forfar and Arneil's Textbook of Paediatrics*, 4th edn, Campbell A.G.M., McIntosh N. (eds). Churchill Livingstone, London, pp. 1047 (1992)

PAK C.Y.C. The spectrum and pathogenesis of hypercalciuria. *Urological Clinics of North America*, **8**, 245–252 (1981)

STARK H., TIEDER M., EINSTEIN B., DAVIDOVITS M. and LITWIN A. Hypercalciuria as a cause of persistent or recurrent haematuria. *Archives of Disease in Childhood*, **63**, 312–313 (1988)

GEARHART J.P., HERZBERG G.I. and JEFF R.D. Childhood urolithiasis: experiences and advances. *Pediatrics*, **87**, 445–450 (1991)

Case 9

Answers

		Score
1.	Pulmonary haemosiderosis.	(+4)
2.	Blood (+2), iron (+2), steroids (+2).	(+6)
		(+10)

Others

Q1: Chronic interstitial pneumonitis (Hamman–Rich syndrome) (+3); Goodpasture's syndrome (+1), polyarteritis nodosum (+1).
Q2: Azathioprine (+0.5).

(Average)

Discussion

This boy had recurrent symptoms of fever, cough and haemoptysis. Investigation showed a microcytic anaemia, a diffuse pulmonary infiltrate and abnormal pulmonary gas exchange. Haemoptysis is an unusual problem in childhood and may follow a pulmonary infection, chemical injury and haemosiderin deposition in the lungs. Primary haemosiderosis may be: (i) an idiopathic condition or is associated with, (ii) cow's milk hypersensitivity, (iii) myocarditis and (iv) Goodpasture's syndrome. Secondary haemosiderosis follows chronic left ventricular failure, mitral stenosis, haemochromatosis and connective tissue disease (e.g. SLE, rheumatoid disease, polyarthritis nodosum). Examination of a sputum sample should reveal the presence of haemosiderin laden macrophages. Further investigations should include an ECG, echocardiogram, assessment of renal function (and a renal biopsy if Goodpasture's syndrome is suspected), and detection of serum antibodies to cow's milk protein. A lung biopsy may be indicated in difficult cases and would show intra-alveolar haemorrhages, haemosiderin laden macrophages, epithelial hyperplasia and fibrosis. Immunoglobulin and complement deposition on the alveolar basement membrane is present in Goodpasture's syndrome. Treatment includes correction of the anaemia and steroids. However, the results of treatment with steroids are variable and they may not be beneficial for some patients.

Further reading

Pulmonary haemosiderosis. In *Nelson Textbook of Pediatrics*, 14th edn, Behrmann R.E. (ed). W.B. Saunders, Philadelphia, pp. 1089–1090 (1992)

Pulmonary haemosiderosis. In *Forfar and Arneil's Textbook of Paediatrics*, 4th edn, Campbell A.G.M., McIntosh N. (eds). Churchill Livingstone, London, pp. 652–653 (1992)

BECKERMAN R.C., TAUSSIG L.M. and PINNAS J.L. Familial idiopathic hemosiderosis. *American Journal of Disease in Childhood*, **133**, 609–611 (1979)

72

SAHA V., RAVIKUMAR E., KHANDURI U., DATE A. and RAGHUPATHY P. Long term prednisolone therapy in children with idiopathic pulmonary hemosiderosis. *Pediatric Haematology and Oncology*, **10**, 89–91 (1992)

Case 10

Answers

		Score
1.	Mucopolysaccharidosis type III (Sanfillipo syndrome).	(+2)
2.	White cell and fibroblast culture and lysosomal enzyme assay (+2); urine heparan, keratan and dermatan sulphate (+2).	(+4)
3.	Hearing aids (+1), ophthalmic review (+1), genetic counselling (+1), behavioural control (+1).	(+4)
		(+10)

Others

Q1: Mucopolysaccharidosis (+1); MPS type VII (+1); GM_1-gangliosidosis (+1); fucosidosis (+1); mannosidosis (+1); sialidosis (+1); Schindler's disease (+1); mucolipidosis I–IV (+1).

Q2: Lateral X-ray of the spine (+1); skeletal survey (+1).

(Average)

Discussion

The family history implied a hereditary condition, probably transmitted in an autosomal recessive fashion. The subsequent clues – deafness, hepatomegaly, behavioural problems and mental retardation – suggested a storage disease and coarse hirsute features with wide metacarpals are typical of the mucopolysaccharidoses. The latter include at least 7 different types. The predominant features in types IV (Morquio's syndrome), IS (Scheie's syndrome) and VI (Maratoux–Lamy syndrome) include marked musculoskeletal deformity and corneal clouding with a relatively normal intellect. Severe musculoskeletal deformity, dwarfism, deafness, and mental retardation is seen in type I (Hurler's syndrome) and II (Hunter's syndrome), though corneal clouding only occurs in Hurler's syndrome. In addition Hunter's syndrome is inherited in an X-linked fashion. Types III (Sanfillipo syndrome) and VII show features spanning both these extremes with moderate musculo-skeletal abnormalities and mental retardation though dwarfism and corneal clouding are rarely seen in these conditions. The specific enzyme defect can be detected by assay of white cell and fibroblast cultures. Mucopolysaccharide metabolites in the form of heparan, keratan and dermatan sulphate can be detected in the urine. A skeletal survey shows the characteristic features of dysostosis multiplex congenita: dolichocephaly; spatulate 'oar-like' ribs; wide diaphyses with narrow epiphyses; wide 'bullet-like' metacarpals, metatarsals and phalanges; hypoplastic acetabulae; kyphoscoliosis; platyvertebrae with anterosuperior ossification defects of the lower vertebral bodies. These radiological appearances can be found in the mucopolysaccharidoses (I–VII), mucolipidoses (I–III) and GM_1 gangliosidosis.

Further reading

The mucopolysaccharidoses. In *Nelson Textbook of Pediatrics*, 14th edn, Behrmann R.E. (ed). W.B. Saunders, Philadelphia, pp. 457, 372–377 (1992)

The mucopolysaccharidoses. In *Forfar and Arneil's Textbook of Paediatrics*, 4th edn, Campbell A.G.M., McIntosh N. (eds). Churchill Livingstone, London, pp. 1241–1244 (1992)

Sanfillipo's syndrome. In *Smith's Recognizable Patterns of Human Malformation*, 4th edn, Jones K.L. (ed). W.B. Saunders, Philadelphia, pp. 414–415 (1988)

DORFMAN A. and MATALON R. The mucopolysaccharidoses (a review). *Proceedings of the National Academy of Science, USA,* **73,** 630–637 (1976)

The mucopolysaccharidoses. In *The Metabolic Basis of Inherited Disease*, 6th edn, Schriver C.W., Beaudet A.L., Sly W.S., Valle D. (eds). Mcgraw Hill, New York, pp. 1565–1588 (1989)

CLEARY M.A. and WRAITH J.E. Management of mucopolysaccharidosis type III. *Archives of Disease in Childhood,* **69,** 403–406 (1993)

Dysostosis multiplex. In *Essentials of Caffey's Pediatric X-ray Diagnosis*, Silverman F.N., Kuhn J.P. (eds). Year Book Medical Publishers, Chicago, pp. 904–910 (1990)

Case 11

Answers

		Score
1.	Werdnig–Hoffmann disease or congenital myopathy.	(+2)
2.	EMG (+1.5), muscle biopsy (+1.5);	(+3)
	nerve conduction tests (+1), septic screen (+1), potassium (+1), glucose (+1), further cranial ultrasound (+1).	(+5)

(+10)

Others

Q1: Meconium aspiration (+1); septicaemia (+1); anoxic-ischaemic damage (+0.5).

(Average)

Discussion

As one reads this case report, the initial impression is that of meconium aspiration in a neonate who may have been asphyxiated during the delivery. However, the initial blood gas and subsequent rapid weaning from the ventilator would contradict this diagnosis. As the story unfolds it becomes clear that this baby was rather 'floppy' with a weak cry, poor sucking reflex and poor respiratory effort. The latter would account for the ensuing respiratory acidosis and atelectasis whilst breathing spontaneously (and rapidly corrected by artificial ventilation). An inability to swallow would account for the polyhydramnios.

The causes for a generally floppy infant at this stage would include severe hypoxic brain disease (particularly involving the cerebellum), hypothyroidism, congenital myasthenia gravis and primary diseases of muscle and nerves. The normal Guthrie test virtually excludes hypothyroidism whereas congenital myasthenia gravis is unlikely in a child born to a normal mother. The absence of deep tendon reflexes is indicative of a primary neuro-muscular abnormality. In this particular case it is likely to be either due to congenital myopathy or Werdnig–Hoffmann disease.

Further reading

Spinal muscular atrophy. In *Nelson Textbook of Pediatrics*, 14th edn, Behrmann R.E. (ed). W.B. Saunders, Philadelphia, pp. 1555 (1992)

Spinal muscular atrophy. In *Forfar and Arneil's Textbook of Paediatrics*, 4th edn, Campbell A.G.M., McIntosh N. (eds). Churchill Livingstone, London, pp. 786 (1992)

Congenital myopathy. In *Nelson Textbook of Pediatrics*, 14th edn, Behrmann R.E. (ed). W.B. Saunders, Philadelphia, pp. 1540 (1992)

Congenital myopathy. In *Forfar and Arneil's Textbook of Paediatrics*, 4th edn, Campbell A.G.M., McIntosh N. (eds). Churchill Livingstone, London, pp. 799–801 (1992)

BARTH P.G., VAN WIJNGAARDEN G.K. and BETHLEM J. X-linked myotubular myopathy with fatal neonatal asphyxia. *Neurology,* **25,** 531–536 (1975)

RUSSMAN B.S., MELCHREIT R. and DRENNAN J.C. Spinal muscular atrophy: the natural course of disease. *Muscle and Nerve,* **6,** 179–181 (1983)

PEARN J. Classification of spinal muscular atrophies. *Lancet,* **i,** 919–921 (1980)

RUTHERFORD M.A., HECKMATT J.Z. and DUBOWITZ V. Congenital myotonic dystrophy: respiratory function at birth determines survival. *Archives of Disease in Childhood,* **64,** 191–195 (1988)

REARDON W., NEWCOMBE R., FENTON I., SIBERT J. and HARPER P.S. The natural history of congenital myotonic dystrophy: mortality and long term clinical aspects. *Archives of Disease in Childhood,* **68,** 177–1 (1993)

Case 12

Answers

		Score
1.	Diurnal serum cortisols (+2);	(+2)
	Overnight dexamethasone suppression test (+1), ultrasound abdomen or CT/MRI abdomen (+1), CT/MRI brain (+1).	(+4)
2.	Cushing's syndrome due to an adrenal tumour or Cushing's disease (pituitary tumour).	(+4)
		(+10)

Others

Q1: Blood glucose (+0.5), adrenocorticotrophic hormone (ACTH) levels (+0.5), 24 hour urine steroid profile (+0.5), investigate urinary tract (+0.5).

(Easy)

Discussion

This girl presented with a urinary tract infection. She was obese for her age and height and had unsightly acne. Both these findings may be normal but, in the presence of systemic hypertension, are indicative of Cushing's syndrome. The most common cause for Cushing's syndrome is treatment with exogenous steroids. Non-iatrogenic causes include a pituitary ACTH-secreting adenoma (Cushing's disease) and an adrenal adenoma or adenocarcinoma. Other steroid hormone secreting tumours are extremely rate. The investigation of this case should therefore include tests aimed at: (a) confirming the abnormal cortisol profile and (b) identifying the most likely source of the abnormal hormone production – a tumour of the pituitary or adrenal gland.

Further reading

Cushing's syndrome. In *Nelson Textbook of Pediatrics*, 14th edn, Behrmann R.E. (ed). W.B. Saunders, Philadelphia, pp. 1448–1450 (1992)

Cushing's syndrome. In *Forfar and Arneil's Textbook of Paediatrics*, 4th edn, Campbell A.G.M., McIntosh N. (eds). Churchill Livingstone, London, pp. 1138 (1992)

HOWLETT T. and BESSER M. Cushing's syndrome. *Medicine International*, **63,** 2605–2611 (1989)

LEE P.D.K., WINTER R.J. and GREEN O.C. Visualising adrenocortical tumours in childhood: eight cases and review of the literature. *Pediatrics*, **76,** 437–444 (1984)

Adrenal steroid excess. In *Clinical Paediatric Endocrinology*, 2nd edn, Brook C.G.D. (ed). Blackwell Scientific, Oxford, pp. 368–406 (1989)

KAYE, T.B. and CRAPO I. The Cushing's syndrome: An update on diagnostic tests. *Annals of Internal Medicine*, **112,** 434–444 (1990)

Case 13

Answers

		Score
1.	Muscle biopsy;	(+2)
	Creatinine phosphokinase (CPK) (+1.5), EMG (+1.5);	(+3)
	antinuclear antibodies (ANA).	(+1)
2.	Dermatomyositis.	(+2)
3.	Steroids and physiotherapy.	(+2)
		(+10)

Others

Q1: Slit lamp examination (+0.5), HLA B8 (+0.5), raised aldolase level (+0.5), LDH (+0.5).
Q2: Systemic lupus erythematosis (SLE) (+1).

(Easy)

Discussion

This boy developed a photosensitive rash, lassitude, pain and weakness of the lower limbs and trunk. A haematological malignancy and infection including HIV and toxoplasmosis may present in this way though the unremarkable investigative results would make these diagnoses less likely. Myopathies, poliomyositis, Guillain–Barré syndrome and myasthenia gravis are not usually associated with skin manifestations. Therefore, the mode of presentation would be in keeping with a connective tissue disorder, especially dermatomyositis, and this is not excluded by a low ESR. The characteristic heliotrope rash around the eyelids and nose is due to a vasculitis of the underlying skin. A similar process results in erythema over the extensor joint surfaces of the knuckles, knees and elbows. The inflammatory process may be associated with areas of local tenderness, oedema, induration (e.g. Gottron pads over knuckles), ulceration and calcinosis. A painful myositis affects the axial and proximal limb muscles, a combination rarely seen in SLE. This myositis may result in profound stiffness and weakness. Indeed some of these children are unable to stand from a sitting position and have to employ a Gower-like manoeuvre not dissimilar to children with muscular dystrophy. The inflammatory process may involve the eyes, joints, lungs, neurological and gastrointestinal tracts. The diagnosis is confirmed on finding elevated serum CPK, aldolase and LDH levels, a moderately elevated ANA level, an EMG showing a myopathic pattern with areas of fibrillation indicative of necrosis, and a muscle biopsy showing perifascicular degeneration and atrophy with an inflammatory cell infiltrate.

Further reading

Dermatomyositis. In *Nelson Textbook of Pediatrics*, 14th edn, Behrmann R.E. (ed). W.B. Saunders, Philadelphia, pp. 632–633 and 1552–1553 (1992)

Dermatomyositis. In *Forfar and Arneil's Textbook of Paediatrics*, 4th edn, Campbell A.G.M., McIntosh N. (eds). Churchill Livingstone, London, pp. 801 and 1681 (1992)

SILVER R.M. and MARICQ H.R. Childhood dermatomyositis. Serial microvascular studies. *Pediatrics*, **83**, 278–283 (1989)

PLOTZ P.H. Current concepts in the idiopathic inflammatory myopathies: polymyositis, dermatomyositis and related disorders. *Annals of Internal Medicine*, **111**, 143–157 (1989)

GOEL K.M. and SHANKS R.A. Dermatomyositis in childhood. *Archives of Disease in Childhood*, **51**, 501–506 (1976)

DE BENEDETTI F., DE AMICI M., ARAMINI L., RUPERTO N. and MARTINI A. Correlation of serum neopterin concentration with disease activity in juvenile dermatomyositis. *Archives of Disease in Childhood*, **69**, 232–235 (1993)

Case 14

Answers

		Score
1.	Barium swallow;	(+2)
	oesophageal pH studies (+1), repeat sweat test (+1), immunoglobulins (+1).	(+3)
2.	Iron deficiency due to oesophageal haemorrhage and chronic infection.	(+2)
3.	Recurrent aspiration secondary to H-type tracheo-oesophageal fistula.	(+3)
		(+10)

Others

Q3: Gastro-oesophageal reflux (+2).

(Average)

Discussion

This infant's failure to thrive is associated with pneumonia (as evidenced by the history, and chronic respiratory signs on examination). There are a number of possible causes of severe, recurrent chest infections in this age group. Cystic fibrosis may present with a similar picture. Strictly speaking there should be more than 100 mg of sweat for the sweat test to be conclusive – nevertheless, the level of sodium in 92 mg of sweat was low and not equivocal, making cystic fibrosis an unlikely diagnosis. Immunodeficiency, in particular IgA deficiency, is also a possibility and the immunoglobulin levels must be quantified. Congenital malformations such as Kartagener's immotile cilia syndrome, bronchial cyst, cystic adenomatous malformation and sequestrated lung are associated with characteristic appearances on the chest X-ray. Recurrent chest infections may also result from aspiration of gastro-oesophageal contents. This is seen in babies with gastro-oesophageal reflux (GOR), oesophageal incoordination syndromes, neurological abnormalities (e.g. pseudobulbar palsy) and tracheo-oesophageal fistulae (TOF). In this infant a barium swallow test carried out in the prone position (i.e. with the trachea dependent relative to the oesophagus) resulted in marked respiratory distress. This position would facilitate the passage of barium into the lungs in the presence of an H-type tracheo-oesophageal fistula. Indeed, this is the only type of TOF that would present after the first few days of life.

Further reading

Gastro-oesophageal reflux. In *Nelson Textbook of Pediatrics*, 14th edn, Behrmann R.E. (ed). W.B. Saunders, Philadelphia, pp. 943–945 (1992)

Gastro-oesophageal reflux. In *Forfar and Arneil's Textbook of Paediatrics*, 4th edn, Campbell A.G.M., McIntosh N. (eds). Churchill Livingstone, London, pp. 495–498 and 1867 (1992)

Tracheo-oesophageal fistula. In *Nelson Textbook of Pediatrics*, 14th edn, Behrmann R.E. (ed). W.B. Saunders, Philadelphia, pp. 941–942 (1992)

Tracheo-oesophageal fistula. In *Forfar and Arneil's Textbook of Paediatrics*, 4th edn, Campbell A.G.M., McIntosh N. (eds). Churchill Livingstone, London, pp. 592 and 1852 (1992)

80

ORENSTEIN S.R. and ORENSTEIN D.M. Gastro-oesophageal reflux and respiratory disease in children. *Journal of Pediatrics,* **112,** 847–858 (1988)

REYES H.M., MELLER J.L. and LOEFF D. Management of oesophageal atresia and tracheo-oesophageal fistula. *Clinical Perinatology,* **16,** 79–84 (1989)

BOOTH I.W. Silent gastro-oesophageal reflux: How much do we miss? *Archives of Disease in Childhood,* **67,** 1325–1327 (1992)

Case 15

Answers

		Score
1.	Treatment of: raised intracranial pressure and seizures (+0.5); pneumonia (+0.5); anaemia (+0.5); hypoglycaemia (+0.5); hyponatraemia (+0.5) and hypokalaemia (+0.5).	(+3)
2.	T-cell subsets (+0.5), immunoglobulins (+0.5), stool and CSF virology (+0.5); blood culture (+0.5), blood gas (+0.5).	(+2.5)
3	Polio vaccine virus encephalitis.	(+2)
4.	Severe combined immunodeficiency.	(+2.5)
		(+10)

Others

Q2: Urine and serum osmolality (+0.25).
Q3: Viral infection (+1).
Q4: Immunodeficiency (+1).

(Hard)

Discussion

This boy presented in status epilepticus with signs of raised intracranial pressure. He had developed a generalized infection involving the central nervous system, the lungs and gastrointestinal tract. A male sibling had died at a similar age, again from overwhelming infection. This suggests an inherited immuno-deficiency syndrome and, since both brothers were affected, probably X-linked recessive in nature. The pattern of infection suggests hypogammaglobulinaemia. However, he also had chronic oral moniliasis, suggestive of T-cell deficiency. All these features together point toward a primary diagnosis of severe combined immunodeficiency (SCID). By the age of 3–6 months transplacentally acquired IgG levels fall. Infants with SCID are unable to produce their own antibody and are no longer protected against severe infection. If so the recent vaccination (including diphtheria and tetanus toxoid and live attenuated poliomyelitis virus) would explain this child's fatal illness due to polio encephalitis. In the UK, childhood poliomyelitis is almost entirely vaccine related and in a child with SCID would result in a fatal infection. Confirmation of the infection is based on the isolation and serotyping of the virus from a stool specimen.

SCID describes a heterogenous group of disorders which include those with X-linked inheritance, adenosine deaminase deficiency and reticular dysgenesis. SCID can be confirmed by demonstrating lymphopenia, agammaglobulinaemia and severely impaired *in vitro* T-cell responses to mitogens. The ideal management would normally involve allogenic HLA-matched bone marrow transplantation, preferably prior to the development of recurrent infection and failure to thrive. Genetic counselling for the families at risk is of paramount importance.

Further reading

Poliomyelitis. In *Nelson Textbook of Pediatrics*, 14th edn, Behrmann R.E. (ed). W.B. Saunders, Philadelphia, pp. 823–832 (1992)

Poliomyelitis. In *Forfar and Arneil's Textbook of Paediatrics*, 4th edn, Campbell A.G.M., McIntosh N. (eds). Churchill Livingstone, London, pp. 1434–1437 (1992)

Severe combined immunodeficiency syndrome. In *Nelson Textbook of Pediatrics*, 14th edn, Behrmann R.E. (ed). W.B. Saunders, Philadelphia, pp. 554–555 (1992)

Severe combined immunodeficiency syndrome. In *Forfar and Arneil's Textbook of Paediatrics*, 4th edn, Campbell A.G.M., McIntosh N. (eds). Churchill Livingstone, London, pp. 1311–1312 (1992)

MELNICH J.L. Advantages and disadvantages of killed and live poliomyelitis vaccine. *Bulletin of the World Health Organisation*, **56**, 21–38 (1978)

WYATT H.V. Risk of live poliomyelitis virus in immunodeficient children. *Journal of Pediatrics*, **87**, 142–153 (1975)

ROSEN F.S., COOPER M.D. and WEDGEWOOD R.J.P. The primary immunodeficiencies. *New England Journal of Medicine*, **311**, 235–242 (part 1) and 300–310 (part 2) (1984)

HERROD H.G. Combined T-cell and B-cell abnormalities. In *Infections in Immunocompromised Infants and Children*. Patrick C.C. (ed). Churchill Livingstone, London, pp. 67–68 (1992)

Case 16

Answers

		Score
1.	Air insufflation enema (barium enema).	(+2)
2.	Intussusception.	(+3)
3.	Neurofibromatosis.	(+3)
4.	Non-Hodgkin's lymphoma.	(+2)
		(+10)

Others

Q1: Homovanyllic acid (HVA) (+0.5), vanyl mandelic acid (VMA) (+0.5), CT abdomen (+0.5).

(Hard)

Discussion

A history of intermittent abdominal pain associated with an abdominal mass which was also intermittently palpable is suggestive of an intussusception. This condition is usually seen in children aged between 1–3 years and is unusual in this age group. This implies that there may have been an underlying abnormality in the gastrointestinal tract acting as the leading focus for the intussusception. Further clues were provided, namely, this boy had a large head, birth marks and skin nodules, features which describe the macrocephaly, café au lait spots and neurofibromas seen in neurofibromatosis type I (NF-1). This condition is known to be associated with an increased risk of developing tumours. In fact this boy had developed a non-Hodgkin's lymphoma. Lymphomatous infiltration can result in the thickening of the intestinal lining which then forms the basis for the intussusceptum.

NF-1 is by far the more common type of neurofibromatosis. The abnormal gene is carried on chromosome 17 as compared with chromosome 22 for NF-2. The two conditions can be distinguished by the features listed in the following table.

NF-1 (90%)	NF-2 (10%)
1. Five or more café au lait spots	1. Bilateral acoustic neuroma.
2. Axillary/inguinal freckling	2. Parent, sibling, child with:
3. Two or more Lisch nodules	– unilateral acoustic neuroma
4. Two or more skin neurofibromas or one plexiform neuroma	3. Parent, sibling or child with 2 of:
5. Optic gliomas	– neurofibromas
6. Osseous lesions:	– meningioma
– kyphoscoliosis	– glioma
– bowed tibia/fibula	– schwannoma
– pseudoarthroses	– posterior lens opacities
– sphenoid dysplasia	
7. First degree relative with 1–6.	

Further reading

Intussusception. In *Nelson Textbook of Pediatrics*, 14th edn, Behrman R.E. (ed). W.B. Saunders, Philadelphia, pp. 958–959 (1992)

Intussusception. In *Forfar and Arneil's textbook of Paediatrics*, 4th edn, Campbell A.G.M., McIntosh N. (eds). Churchill Livingstone, London, pp. 1867–1868 (1992)

REIJNEN J.A.M., FESTEN C. and VAN ROOSMALEN R.P. Intussusception: factors related to treatment. *Archives of Disease in Childhood,* **65,** 871–873 (1990)

DEN HOLLANDER D. and BARGE D.M. Exclusion criteria and outcome in pressure reduction of intussusception. *Archives of Disease in Childhood,* **68,** 79–81 (1993)

Neurofibromatosis. In *Nelson Textbook of Pediatrics*, 14th edn, Behrman R.E. (ed). W.B. Saunders, Philadelphia, pp. 1509–1510 (1992)

Neurofibromatosis. In *Forfar and Arneil's Textbook of Paediatrics*, 4th edn, Campbell A.G.M., McIntosh N. (eds). Churchill Livingstone, London, pp. 874–901 (1992)

Neurofibromatosis. In *Smith's Recognizable Patterns of Human Malformation,* 4th edn, Jones K.L. (ed). W.B. Saunders, Philadelphia, pp. 452–453 (1988)

LISTERNICH R. and CHARROW J. Neurofibromatosis type 1 in Childhood. *Journal of Pediatrics,* **116,** 845–853 (1990)

BERRY C.L. and KEELING J.W. Gastrointestinal lymphoma in childhood. *Journal of Clinical Pathology,* **23,** 459–463 (1970)

Case 17

Answers

		Score
1.	Wilson's disease.	(+2)
2.	Serum caeruloplasmin (+1); urine copper excretion (+1); slit lamp examination (+1); copper content on liver biopsy (+1); assess ^{64}Cu uptake (+1).	(+5)
3.	Chelation treatment with D-penicillamine or TETA (+2); liver transplantation (+1).	(+3)
		(+10)

Others

Q2: Serum copper (+0.5), liver ultrasound (+0.5).

(Hard)

Discussion

This child presented with neurological symptoms and signs suggestive of a problem with the basal ganglia. In addition the hypoalbuminaemia, abnormal liver enzymes and hepatomegaly are indicative of liver dysfunction. These findings in the same patient can be explained by Wilson's disease – also known as hepatolenticular degeneration. The condition is inherited as an autosomal recessive trait, and is due to the presence of defective copper binding proteins. Unbound copper spills into the circulation and is deposited in several organs. The excess copper accumulation causes liver damage ranging from mild fatty change (with asymptomatic hepatomegaly), to hepatitis, cirrhosis and portal hypertension. Neurological sequelae occur in 20% of patients and follow copper deposition in the basal ganglia and lentiform nuclei. This may result in a tremor, dystonia, speech disabilities, parkinsonian gait, behavioural problems and decreased school performance. Ophthalmic involvement results in Kayser–Fleischer rings which are usually not seen before 7 years of age. Copper-induced haemolysis, arthritis, renal failure and a renal Fanconi-like tubular acidosis are other complications. Those patients with significant liver disease tend to present earlier (4–8 years), whereas neurological features are typical of older patients. Laboratory diagnosis is based on the confirmation of a low caeruloplasmin level, excess copper deposition on liver biopsy and increased urinary copper excretion. The latter is enhanced following a loading dose of penicillamine. Serum copper levels are usually low. In equivocal cases a definitive diagnosis can be made by assessing the uptake and excretion of radiolabelled ^{64}Cu. Treatment entails copper chelation with D-penicillamine or triethylene tetramine hydrochloride (TETA). Treatment is most effective if commenced early and therefore prompt screening of siblings is essential.

Further reading

Wilson's disease. In *Nelson Textbook of Pediatrics*, 14th edn, Behrman R.E. (ed). W.B. Saunders, Philadelphia, pp. 1015–1016 (1992)

Wilson's disease. In *Forfar and Arneil's Textbook of Paediatrics*, 4th edn, Campbell A.G.M., McIntosh N. (eds). Churchill Livingstone, London, pp. 554–555, 826–830, 892 and 1213 (1992)

DUBOIS R.S., RODGERSON D.O. and HAMBIDGE K.M. Treatment of Wilson's disease with triethylene tetramine hydrochloride. *Journal of Pediatric Gastroenterology and Nutrition,* **10**, 77–81 (1990)

NAZER H., EDE R.J., MOWAT A.P. and WILLIAM R. Wilson's disease: clinical presentation and use of prognostic index. *Gut,* **27**, 1377–1381 (1986)

Wilson's disease. In *The Metabolic Basis of Inherited Disease*, 6th edn, Schriver C.W., Beaudet A.L., Sly W.S., Valle D. (eds). McGraw Hill, New York, pp. 1416–1421 (1989)

Case 18

Answers

		Score
1.	Reactive arthropathy with effusions;	(+1.5)
	Bone cyst/tumour of the upper fibula (discovered incidentally).	(+1.5)
2.	Stool cultures (+1), culture effusion fluid (+1), serum antibodies for yersinia, shigella, salmonella, pathological *E. coli*, entero-viruses (+1).	(+3)
	Initial bed rest (+0.5), analgesics (+0.5), aspirate tense effusions (+0.5), physiotherapy (+0.5).	(+2)
	Biopsy fibula.	(+2)
		(+10)

Others

Q2: Skeletal survey (+0.5), bone scan (+0.5).

(Easy)

Discussion

The history in this case was that of a boy who developed a reactive arthropathy following a bout of food poisoning. Similar problems generally follow infection with salmonella, shigellae, campylobacter and yersinia. Affected individuals are often HLA B27 positive. The arthropathy, though painful and incapacitating, is almost always transient and non-deforming. A single or a small number of large joints is usually affected. Aspiration of a joint reveals cloudy effusion fluid with an increased white cell count, mostly polymorphs, slightly decreased glucose levels compared with the serum level and no organisms on microscopy or culture. The treatment is supportive with analgesics and mobilisation plus physiotherapy as soon as this can be tolerated by the patient.

The lesion in the fibula had a periosteal reaction and was therefore present for some time. Furthermore, bone 'cysts' are not a feature of a reactive arthropathy. This was an incidental finding and merits investigation separately – with a biopsy in the first instance as the radiological appearance, though atypical, did not rule out a malignant lesion.

Further reading

Reactive arthropathy. In *Nelson Textbook of Pediatrics*, 14th edn, Behrman R.E. (ed).
W.B. Saunders, Philadelphia, pp. 623, 695–698 and 730 (1992)

KUNNAMO I., KALLIO P., PELKONEN P. and HOVI T. Clinical signs and laboratory tests in the differential diagnosis of arthritis in children. *American Journal of Disease in Childhood*, **141**, 34–40 (1987)

COHEN J.I., BARTLETT J.A. and COREZ G.R. Extra-intestinal manifestations of salmonella infections. *Medicine*, **66**, 349–388 (1987)

Case 19

Answers

		Score
1.	Fanconi's anaemia.	(+2)
2.	White cell chromosome fragility tests.	(+2)
3.	Acute (myeloid) leukaemia.	(+2)
4.	Supportive antibiotics (+1), blood (+1), platelet transfusions (+1), chemotherapy (+1).	(+4)

(+10)

Others

Q4: Bone marrow transplant (+0.5).

(Hard)

Discussion

Acute leukaemia must be considered when this child presented at the age of four with bruises and bone pain and was found to have generalized lymphadenopathy, hepatosplenomegaly, anaemia and thrombocytopenia with a raised white cell count. A hypercellular bone marrow with sheets of blast cells is typical of this condition. Bony irregularities on X-ray are not uncommon and due to local infiltration and destruction by leukaemic cells. In this child the leukaemia followed a previous history of bone marrow dysfunction and indeed, pancytopenia was noted at the age of 2 years. In addition this child was physically small with dysmorphic features including abnormal thumbs and hyperpigmentation, a combination indicative of a congenital aplastic anaemia particularly of the Fanconi type. The pancytopenia is often associated with a red cell macrocytosis and an increase in fetal haemoglobin. Fanconi's anaemia, like xeroderma pigmentosum and Bloom's syndrome, is one of the chromosome fragility syndromes. All these conditions carry a greatly increased risk for developing malignant disease, especially of haematological origins. The diagnosis of Fanconi anaemia can be made by demonstrating a 50–200 times increase in chromosomal breaks, exchanges and bizarre rearrangements following exposure to mitomycin C, nitrogen mustards or diepoxy-butane (DEB). It is inherited as a recessive condition with variable penetrance.

Further reading

Fanconi's Anaemia. In *Nelson Textbook of Pediatrics*, 14th edn, Behrman R.E. (ed). W.B. Saunders, Philadelphia, pp. 1528 (1992)

Fanconi's Anaemia. In *Forfar and Arneil's Textbook of Paediatrics*, 4th edn, Campbell A.G.M., McIntosh N. (eds). Churchill Livingstone, London, pp. 925 (1992)

Fanconi's Anaemia. In *Smith's Recognizable Patterns of Human Malformation*, 4th edn, Jones K.L. (ed). W.B. Saunders, Philadelphia, pp. 274–275 (1988)

ALTER B.P. and POTTER N.U. Classification and aetiology of the aplastic anaemias. *Clinical Haematology*, **7**, 431–466 (1978)

BLOOM G.E., WARNER S., GERALD B.S. and DIAMOND L.K. Chromosome abnormalities in constitutional aplastic anaemia. *New England Journal of Medicine*, **274**, 8–14 (1966)

SWIFT M.R. and HIRSCHHORN K. Fanconi's Anaemia. *Annals of Internal Medicine*, **65**, 496–503 (1966)

Case 20

Answers

		Score
1.	Acute on chronic pancreatitis with pseudocyst.	(+3)
2.	Serum amylase (+1), immunoreactive trypsin (IRT) (+1), abdominal ultrasound (serial) (+1), abdominal CT scan (+1).	(+4)
3.	Restrict oral intake (+0.5), intravenous fluids (+0.5), TPN (+0.5), blood transfusion (+0.5), analgesics (+0.5), drain pseudocyst (+0.5).	(+3)
		(+10)

Others

Q1: Neuroblastoma (+0.5), vasoactive intestinal peptide (VIP) secreting tumour (+0.5), non-Hodgkin's lymphoma (NHL) (+0.5), nephroblastoma (+0.5), retroperitoneal sarcoma (+0.5), abdominal tuberculosis (+0.5).

Q2: Clotting profile (+0.5), urinary VMA and HMA (+0.5), sweat test (+0.5).

(Hard)

Discussion

This boy had a history of abdominal pain and presented acutely with an ileus, an abdominal mass and signs of a left-sided pleural effusion. An acute haemorrhage into an existing abdominal mass may be associated with an ileus, and the differential diagnosis should include abdominal lymphoma, neuroblastoma and nephroblastoma. The latter two conditions may show areas of calcification within a soft tissue mass on an abdominal X-ray. However, the length of the history was against a diagnosis of malignant disease, and these tumours are more likely to produce gastrointestinal obstruction rather than an ileus. A 'benign' vasoactive intestinal peptide (VIP) secreting tumour may have accounted for the bouts of abdominal pain and loose stools. Abdominal tuberculosis generally results in ascites and a non-central mass. None of these conditions would explain the metabolic derangements observed in this case.

Pancreatitis and pseudocyst formation is uncommon in the paediatric age group. Children with pancreatitis are often toxic and in considerable pain. They resist any movement and, particularly with haemorrhagic pancreatitis, may develop bruising over the flanks (Grey Turner sign). The condition may be idiopathic or follow abdominal trauma, drugs, toxins and systemic viral infection. Recurrent pancreatitis may be associated with cystic fibrosis, hereditary autosomal dominant chronic pancreatitis, hyperlipidaemia, hyperparathyroidism and α_1-antitrypsin deficiency. The diagnosis may be confirmed by finding raised serum amylase and immunoreactive trypsin (IRT) levels, and abdominal imaging. Attention should be paid to pain control and nutrition. Patients should be strictly nil by mouth and parenteral nutrition started early in severe cases. Most small pseudocysts resolve spontaneously. Larger ones may require drainage (percutaneously in experienced hands), preferably after 4 weeks, by which time the pseudocyst should have become walled off.

Further reading

Pancreatitis. In *Nelson Textbook of Pediatrics*, 14th edn, Behrman R.E. (ed). W.B. Saunders, Philadelphia, pp. 998–1000 (1992)

Pancreatitis. In *Forfar and Arneil's Textbook of Paediatrics*, 4th edn, Campbell A.G.M., McIntosh N. (eds). Churchill Livingstone, London, pp. 520 (1992)

JORDAN S.C. and AMENT M.E. Pancreatitis in children and adolescence. *Journal of Pediatrics*, **91**, 211–216 (1977)

WEIZMAN Z. and DURIE P.R. Acute pancreatitis in childhood. *Journal of Pediatrics*, **113**, 24–29 (1988)

MILLAR A.J., RODE H., STUNDEN R.J. and CYMES S. Management of pancreatic pseudocyst in children. *Journal of Pediatric Surgery*, **23**, 122–127 (1988)

Pancreatitis. In *Pediatric Gastrointestinal Disease*, Walker W.A., Durie P.R., Amilton J.R., Walker-Smith J.A., Watkin J.B. (eds). B.C. Becker, pp. 1201–1234 (1991)

Case 21

Answers

		Score
1.	Maternal drug abuse (opiates).	(+5)
2.	Control fits with diazepam, followed by high dose chlorpromazine.	(+5)
		(+10)

Others

Q1: Maternal alcohol consumption (+2).

(Average)

Discussion

This case centres around the differential diagnosis of early neo-natal convulsions. Some causes could be excluded from the history and the apparently normal examination – namely birth asphyxia, trauma and congenital or chromosomal defects. The investigative results would argue against hypo/hypernatraemia, hypocalcaemia, hypomagnesaemia, hyperphosphataemia and hypoglycaemia as causes for the fits. Despite the family history, inborn errors of metabolism are likely to be associated with a significant metabolic acidosis and, in the case of the urea cycle defects, with significant hyperammonaemia. Furthermore there was no evidence for infection on the peripheral blood count and microscopy of the CSF. This leaves withdrawal fits secondary to maternal drug abuse as the most likely diagnosis. Most abused drugs cross the placenta and can cause withdrawal problems in up to 75% of babies. Heroin and methadone are the usual offenders though similar problems arise with benzodiazepines, barbiturates and cocaine. The affected baby usually presents with a tremor and irritability, though poor feeding, tachypnoea, nasal congestion, yawning, diarrhoea and convulsions are among other less common symptoms of the neonatal drug withdrawal syndrome. Treatment can be difficult and generally involves heavy sedation, occasionally with massive doses of chlorpromazine, until seizure control is achieved. The dose is then gradually reduced and discontinued over a prolonged period.

Further reading

Opiate withdrawal. In *Nelson Textbook of Pediatrics*, 14th edn, Behrman R.E. (ed). W.B. Saunders, Philadelphia, pp. 490–491 and 1500–1501 (1992)

NEUMANN L.L. and COHEN S.N. The neonatal narcotic withdrawal syndrome. *Clinics in Perinatology*, **2**, 99–109 (1975)

HERZLINGER R.A., KANDALL S.R. and VAUGHAN H.G. Neonatal seizures associated with narcotic withdrawal. *Journal of Pediatrics*, **91**, 638–641 (1977)

MIZRAHI E.M. Neonatal seizures: problems in diagnosis and classification. *Epilepsia*, **28**, 546–555 (1987)

VOLPE J.J. Neonatal seizures: Current concepts and revised classification. *Pediatrics*, **84**, 422–428 (1989)

Case 22

Answers

		Score
1.	ECG to confirm the supraventricular tachycardia (+1), echocardiogram (+1), chest X-ray (+1).	(+3)
2.	Maternal digoxin or flecanide (+1), close follow-up and planned delivery (+1), drain severe pleural effusions and ascites (+1).	(+3)
3.	Ice-cold flannel to face or cold water down nasogastric tube (+1), adenosine (+1), digoxin or beta-blocker or flecanide (+1), transfuse (+1).	(+4)
		(+10)

Others

Q1: TORCH screen (+0.5), fundoscopy (+0.5), skeletal survey (+0.5), chromosomal analysis (+0.5), renal ultrasound (+0.5).

(Average)

Discussion

This baby was hydropic, in cardiac failure and in respiratory distress. The case centres around the possible causes for hydrops foetalis. The tachypnoea could be explained by a congenital malformation (e.g. adenomatoid cyst or diaphragmatic hernia) or a pneumonitis associated with congenital infection, though there is little evidence for these diagnoses in the case report. Pulmonary oedema and pleural effusions are commonly found in hydropic neonates in cardiac failure, and would have accounted for the pulmonary signs. Congenital infection cannot be discounted: the antenatal history (of a rash/maternal illness) was unavailable, though we were told that the mother was rubella antibody negative. However, rubella is not commonly associated with hydrops (as compared with CMV, syphilis, toxoplasmosis and leptospirosis) and this child did not have splenomegaly or thrombocytopenia. Anaemia is common in severely hydropic neonates and is not necessarily indicative of *in utero* haemolysis. This child's blood group was O-positive making ABO incompatibility unlikely, and rhesus disease of this severity is unusual in a primigravida (who was not known to have had any invasive procedures or placental bleeding in the antenatal period). In view of the presence of a single umbilical artery and hydrops, both a renal ultrasound scan and chromosomal analysis would be justified. However, the most impressive abnormality was the tachycardia, which cannot be explained by failure alone. Indeed, this baby had severe cardiac failure causing hydrops as a result of a supraventricular tachy-arrhythmia (SVT). The management would involve an attempt to reverse the SVT *in utero*, and if this failed, as soon as possible postnatally. Refractory SVT may require a prolonged period of intensive care and carries a high risk of death from cardiac failure and secondary sepsis.

Further reading

Hydrops fetalis. In *Nelson Textbook of Pediatrics*, 14th edn, Behrman R.E. (ed). W.B. Saunders, Philadelphia, pp. 483 (1992)

Hydrops fetalis. In *Forfar and Arneil's Textbook of Paediatrics*, 4th edn, Campbell A.G.M., McIntosh N. (eds). Churchill Livingstone, London, pp. 257–259 (1992)

Supraventricular tachycardia. In *Nelson Textbook of Pediatrics*, 14th edn, Behrman R.E. (ed). W.B. Saunders, Philadelphia, pp. 1193–1196 (1992)

Supraventircular tachycardia. In *Forfar and Arneil's Textbook of Paediatrics*, 4th edn, Campbell A.G.M., McIntosh N. (eds). Churchill Livingstone, London, pp. 696–697 (1992)

CASTILLO R.A., DEVOE C.D., HADI H.A., MARTIN S. and GEIST D. Non immune hydrops fetalis: clinical experience and factors associated with poor outcome. *American Journal of Obstetrics and Gynecology*, **155**, 812–816 (1986)

HOLZGREVE W., CURRY C.R., GOLBUS M.S., CALLEN P.W., FILLEY R.A. and SMITH J.C. Investigation of non-immune hydrops fetalis. *American Journal of Obstetrics and Gynecology*, **150**, 805–812 (1984)

Case 23

Answers

		Score
1.	Folate deficiency.	(+3)
2.	Jejunal biopsy and aspirate.	(+3)
3.	Coeliac disease (+2) and giardiasis (+2).	(+4)
		(+10)

(Hard)

Discussion

This boy's symptoms were progressive weight loss with recurrent diarrhoea. Investigations showed evidence of malabsorption, i.e. an abnormal xylose tolerance test and an increase in the 3 day faecal fat content. The relative eosinophilia was not of the order seen with worm infestation. In children the presence of ova in the stool is common and is often due to localized, rectal *Enterobious vermicularis*. Though resulting in local irritation, the latter is not a cause of malabsorption. Coeliac disease and infection of the small intenstine with *Giardia lamblia* are the two most likely explanations for this boy's malabsorption. In coeliac disease anaemia is common and usually due to iron deficiency though a macrocytic anaemia due to folate deficiency is also possible. Hypoalbuminaemia and reduced gammaglobulin levels occur in up to one third of patients with coeliac disease. A jejunal biopsy and examination of the mucosal lining and aspirate is the best way of clarifying the diagnosis.

Further reading

Coeliac disease. In *Nelson Textbook of Pediatrics*, 14th edn, Behrman R.E. (ed). W.B. Saunders, Philadelphia, pp. 977–979 (1992)

Coeliac disease. In *Forfar and Arneil's Textbook of Paediatrics*, 4th edn, Campbell A.G.M., McIntosh N. (eds). Churchill Livingstone, London, pp. 507–509 (1992)

MCNEISH A.S., HARMS H.K., REY J., *et al.* The diagnosis of coeliac disease – a commentary on the current practise of members of the European Society of Paediatric Gastronenterology and Nutrition. *Archives of Disease in Childhood*, **54**, 783–786 (1979)

WALKER-SMITH J.A. Coeliac Disease. In *Diseases of the Small Intestine in Childhood*. Butterworths, London, pp. 88–143 (1988)

Report to Working Group of European Society of Paediatric Gastroenterology and Nutrition: Revised criteria for the diagnosis of Coeliac Disease. *Archives of Disease in Childhood*, **65**, 909–911 (1990)

THOMAS A.G., PHILLIPS A.D. and WALKER-SMITH J.A. The value of proximal small intestinal biopsy in the differential diagnosis of chronic diarrhoea. *Archives of Disease in Childhood*, **67**, 741–744 (1992)

CATASSI C., RATSCH I-M., FABIANI E., ROSSINI M., BORDICCHIA F., CANDELA F., COPPA G.V. and GIORGI P.L. Coeliac disease in the year 2000: exploring the iceberg. *Lancet*, **343**, 200–203 (1994)

Coeliac disease. In *Diseases of the Small Intestine in Childhood*, 3rd edn, Walker-Smith J.A. (ed). Butterworth, London, pp. 88–135 (1988)

Coeliac disease. In *Pediatric Gastrointestinal Disease*, Walker W.A., Durie P.R., Amilton J.R., Walker-Smith J.A., Watkin J.B. (eds). B.C. Becker, pp. 700–715 (1991).

Case 24

Answers

		Score
1.	Fabry's disease (angiokeratosis corporis diffusum).	(+2)
2.	Ophthalmic review (+1), urine chromatography (for maltese crosses) (+1), bone marrow for foamy cells (+1), leucocyte or fibroblast α-galactosidase assay (+1).	(+4)
3.	Genetic counselling and antenatal screening.	(+2)
4.	Phenytoin for shooting pains.	(+2)

(+10)

(Average)

Discussion

The combination of neurological signs, often worse after exertion, a distinctive rash consisting of dark papules in the bathing trunk area, and proteinuria is suggestive of Fabry's disease. Despite the X-linked recessive inheritance, females may be mildly affected by this condition. The disorder is due to α-galactosidase deficiency which can be confirmed on white cell and skin fibroblast cultures. The enzyme defect results in an excess glycosphingolipid which is deposited in the urine as complexes in the shape of maltese crosses and in the vascular endothelium. Blood vessels supplying the peripheral nerves, the myocardium and kidneys are predominantly affected. This results in an altered sensation and shooting pains along the distribution of peripheral nerves, heart disease and eventually renal failure. Symptoms generally manifest by late childhood and the disease progresses, leading to death from cardiac or renal complications in early adulthood. Though phenytoin may alleviate the limb pains, the management is generally supportive and should include genetic counselling. The differential diagnosis would include other lysosomal storage diseases which may present with a similar rash – fucosidosis, mannosidosis, sialidosis and Schindler's disease.

Further reading

Fabry's disease. In *Nelson Textbook of Pediatrics*, 14th edn, Behrman R.E. (ed). W.B. Saunders, Philadelphia, pp. 348–349 (1992)

Fabry's disease. In *Forfar and Arneil's Textbook of Paediatrics*, 4th edn, Campbell A.G.M., McIntosh N. (eds). Churchill Livingstone, London, pp. 1232 (1992)

Fabry's syndrome. In *Smith's Recognizable Patterns of Human Malformation*, 4th edn, Jones K.L. (ed). W.B. Saunders, Philadelphia, pp. 540–541 (1988)

Fabry's disease: α galactosidase deficiency. In *The Metabolic Basis of Inherited Disease*, 6th edn, Schriver C.W., Beaudet A.L., Sly W.S., Valle D. (eds). McGraw Hill, New York, pp. 1751–1779 (1989)

Case 25

Answers

		Score
1.	Acute glaucoma.	(+3)
2.	Retinoblastoma.	(+3)
3.	Urgent EUA.	(+4)

(+10)

Others

Q2: Ocular toxocariasis (+2).
Q3: Eosinophil count (+1), toxocara antibodies (+1).

(Easy)

Discussion

There are several causes for an absent red reflex but most of these conditions are exceedingly rare in childhood. They include retino-blastoma (producing a white reflex or leukocoria), ocular toxo-cariasis, cataract formation, retinal detachment and vitreous haemorrhage. The last two conditions are generally associated with trauma, bleeding diathesis or retinal diseases including retinoblas-toma. Toxocariasis is acquired from dogs (toxocara canis) or cats (toxocara catis) either by direct contact with infected pets (particu-larly puppies and lactating bitches) or because of pica. Younger children usually develop generalized infection with systemic mani-festations including a fever, respiratory symptoms, seizures, hepatomegaly, skin rashes and lymphadenopathy. Ocular toxo-cariasis, on the other hand, is a disease of older children and is rarely associated with other systemic manifestations. Patients present with decreased acuity in the affected eye, and occasionally with periorbital oedema. The lesions are usually sited towards the back of the orbit around the optic nerve and macula and acute glaucoma is therefore unlikely. In contrast, advanced retinoblas-toma may well disrupt the flow of vitreous humour resulting in painful buphthalmos and periorbital oedema. Most retinoblastomas (approximately 85%) are sporadic and present in children aged 1–3 years. The hereditary forms are inherited in a dominant fashion, are often bilateral and present in younger children (average age 14 months). Screening of siblings with a positive family history allows for the detection of these tumours at an early age. Any child with leukocoria requires urgent specialist referral for an examination under anaesthesia.

Further reading

Retinoblastoma. In *Nelson Textbook of Pediatrics*, 14th edn, Behrman R.E. (ed). W.B. Saunders, Philadelphia, pp. 1314–1315 and 1589–1590 (1992)

Retinoblastoma. In *Forfar and Arneil's Textbook of Paediatrics*, 4th edn, Campbell A.G.M., McIntosh N. (eds). Churchill Livingstone, London, pp. 1750–1751 (1992)

Retinoblastoma. In *Principles and Practise of Pediatric Oncology*. Pizzo P.A., Poplack D.G. (eds). Lippincott, Philadelphia, pp. 555–568 (1989)

DRAPER G.J., SANDERS B.M., BROWNBILL P.A. and HAWKINS M.M. Patterns of risk of hereditary retinoblastoma and applications to genetic counselling. *British Journal of Cancer,* **66,** 211–219 (1992)

SANDERS B.M., DRAPER G.J. and KINGSTON J.E. Retinoblastoma in Great Britain 1969–1980: incidence, treatment and survival. *British Journal of Ophthalmology,* **72,** 576–583 (1988)

Case 26

Answers

		Score
1.	Detailed observation on ward,	(+3)
	in depth discussion with family,	(+2)
	in depth discussion with school,	(+2)
	referral to child psychiatric team.	(+3)
		(+10)

Others

Q1: Repeat MRI scan of brain (+1), EEG during 'fit' (+1), CSF for xanthochromia (+1).

(Easy)

Discussion

Convulsions are rarely a presenting symptom in children with a brain tumour. However, severe headaches, particularly those with a diurnal pattern, should raise the suspicion of an intracranial space occupying lesion, despite the absence of any abnormal physical sign. Indeed this diagnosis was considered but the appropriate, contrasted CT scan was normal. A normal EEG does not rule out intracranial pathology but makes it less likely. On careful assessment of this case certain discrepancies come to light: How did the patient manage to reach the end of the ward (and have a fit?) when she was supposedly unable to walk? Indeed were the symptoms 'genuine', or were they a means to attract attention? This child was the youngest in a large family, was alone at home with (presumably) elderly parents and expected to 'achieve' academically. Was the absenteeism from school anything to do with her marked obesity? Was it a coincidence that she developed 'neurological problems' or did the tragic death of a brother from a subarachnoid haemorrhage have anything to do with this? Certainly several questions remain unanswered, and a referral to a sympathetic child psychologist would be appropriate.

Further reading

Psychosomatic Illness. In *Nelson Textbook of Pediatrics*, 14th edn, Behrman R.E. (ed). W.B. Saunders, Philadelphia, pp. 57 (1992)

Psychosomatic Illness. In *Forfar and Arneil's Textbook of Paediatrics*, 4th edn, Campbell A.G.M., McIntosh N. (eds). Churchill Livingstone, London, pp. 1815 (1992)

GOODYER I. Hysterical conversion reactions in childhood. *Journal of Childhood Psychology and Psychiatry,* **22,** 179–188 (1981)

Case 27

Answers

		Score
1.	Blood cultures, abdominal ultrasound scan.	(+4)
2.	Liver/sub-diaphragmatic abscess.	(+2)
3.	Type Ib glycogen storage disease.	(+4)
		(+10)

Others

Q1: Blood film (+1), anti-neutrophil antibodies (+1).
Q3: Glycogen storage disease (+2).

(Hard)

Discussion

As well as inflammatory bowel disease this boy suffered with recurrent infections. On this occasion he presented with a temperature and drowsiness, developed spiking fevers and had focal signs in the right upper quadrant. A soft tissue mass beneath the area of maximum tenderness was seen on X-ray, raising the possibility of an abscess. Despite his toxic state, investigation showed a relative neutropenia as well as hypoglycaemia. Chronic hepatomegaly and recurrent hypoglycaemia (note the overnight nasogastric feeding), are characteristic of some of the glycogen storage diseases (GSD). In GSD I there is an inability to mobilize glucose from glycogen, resulting in recurrent hypoglycaemic episodes. Lactic acidosis results from the alternative breakdown of glycogen to pyruvate. In addition, in type Ib GSD the metabolic defect also affects leucocytes. Chemotaxis and phagocytosis are defective and the neutrophil count is reduced, rendering these patients highly susceptible to recurrent bacterial infection. Inflammatory bowel disease has been reported to be associated with this inborn error of metabolism.

Further reading

Glycogen Storage disease. In *Nelson Textbook of Pediatrics*, 14th edn, Behrman R.E. (ed). W.B. Saunders, Philadelphia, pp. 365–371 (1992)

Glycogen Storage disease. In *Forfar and Arneil's Textbook of Paediatrics*, 4th edn, Campbell A.G.M., McIntosh N. (eds). Churchill Livingstone, London, pp. 1215–1220 (1992)

BURCHELL A., JUNG R.T., LANG C.C., BENNETT W. and SHEPHERD A.M. Diagnosis of type Ia and Ic Glycogen storage diseases in adults. *Lancet*, **i,** 1059–1062 (1987)

MCADAMS A.J., HUG G. and BORE K.F. Glycogen Storage Disease type I-X: Criteria for morphologic diagnosis. *Human Pathology*, **5,** 463–487 (1974)

Case 28

Answers

Score

1. Pneumonia (+1) and septicaemia (+1) due to
   Streptococcus pneumoniae (+2). (+4)
2. Resuscitate with plasma expanders; i.v. penicillin. (+4)
3. Haemoglobin electrophoresis (+1); complement
   levels (+1). (+2)

   ───────

   (+10)

Others

Q3: Osmotic fragility test (+0.5).

(Average)

Discussion

This girl presented with a lobar pneumonia and, following a delay in the diagnosis and treatment, developed septic shock. Encapsulated strains of *Streptococcus pneumoniae* (especially type 3) are the commonest bacterial cause of lobar pneumonia in western countries (with a peak of 13–18 months). The organism is generally carried in the upper respiratory tract in the majority of healthy individuals. A *Strep. pneumoniae* respiratory tract infection, if left untreated, may result in septicaemia which is associated with a characteristic elevation in the neutrophil count. Those at particular risk of septicaemia include children with haemoglobinopathies (e.g. sickle cell disease), hereditary spherocytosis, asplenia or post splenectomy, nephrotic syndrome, HIV infection and complement deficiencies. Treatment is with penicillin, though an increasing number of penicillin-resistant strains have now been reported. Anti-pneumococcal vaccines cover a limited number of possible pathogenic strains. They generally produce a suboptimal antibody response in children aged less than 2 years. Their use should be limited to those children at risk of developing pneumococcal septicaemia, and be given in addition to long term penicillin prophylaxis. This would apply to the patient in this report who was black, anaemic and had a family history of pneumococcal septicaemia, and was therefore likely to have had sickle cell disease.

Further reading

Streptococcus pneumoniae. In *Nelson Textbook of Pediatrics*, 14th edn, Behrman R.E. (ed). W.B. Saunders, Philadelphia, pp. 709–711 (1992)

Streptococcus pneumoniae. In *Forfar and Arneil's Textbook of Paediatrics*, 4th edn, Campbell A.G.M., McIntosh N. (eds). Churchill Livingstone, London, pp. 642, 1342 and 1374 (1992)

PATON J.C., TOOGOOD I.R., COCKINGTON R.A. and HANSMAN D. Antibody response to pneumococcal vaccine in children aged 5–15 years. *American Journal of Disease in Children,* **140,** 135–138 (1986)

BJORNSON A.B. and LOBEL J.S. Direct evidence that decreased serum opsonisation of streptococcus pneumoniae via the alternative complement pathway in sickle cell disease is related to antibody deficiency. *Journal of Clinical Investigation,* **79,** 388–398 (1987)

Editorial. Pneumonia in childhood. *Lancet,* **i,** 741–743 (1988)

MCLELLAN D. and GIEBINK G.S. Perspectives on occult bacteraemia in children. *Journal of Pediatrics,* **109,** 1–8 (1986)

Case 29

Answers

		Score
1.	Abdominal X-ray (plain and decubitus);	(+2)
	blood glucose (+1), blood culture (+1).	(+2)
2.	Volume replacement (+0.5) with K^+ supplements (+0.5); i.v. antibiotics (+0.5); nil by mouth and nasogastric aspiration (+0.5); cross-match (+0.5) prior to surgery (+0.5).	(+3)
3.	Small bowel volvulus/malrotation.	(+3)
		(+10)

Others

Q1: Urine/stool culture (+0.5).
Q3: Small bowel obstruction (+1).

(Easy)

Discussion

The crux of this question lies in the description of the vomitus – bile stained vomiting implies small intestinal obstruction until proven otherwise. This is particularly the case with high obstructions where abdominal distention may be absent and faeces may still be passed normally. The metabolic acidosis would be expected in a sick infant with gastrointestinal obstruction for this length of time, and is characteristic of high obstructions where there is loss of alkaline vomitus. Sodium and potassium loss into the bowel lumen results in hyponatraemia and hypokalaemia. Pyloric stenosis classically produces a hypochloraemic metabolic alkalosis due to loss of acidic gastric juice, and hypokalaemia due to exchange of K^+ for H^+ ions in the renal tubules. Since the problem arose some time after birth a duodenal or small bowel atresia is unlikely, and the obstruction is probably due to a volvulus secondary to a malrotation of the bowel. These cases require urgent resuscitation and surgical intervention.

Further reading

Small bowel volvulus. In *Nelson Textbook of Pediatrics*, 14th edn, Behrman R.E. (ed). W.B. Saunders, Philadelphia, pp. 951–952 (1992)

Small bowel volvulus. In *Forfar and Arneil's Textbook of Paediatrics*, 4th edn, Campbell A.G.M., McIntosh N. (eds). Churchill Livingstone, London, pp. 856 (1992)

FILSTON H. and KIRKS D.R. Malrotation – the ubiquitous anomaly. *Journal of Pediatric Surgery*, **16,** 614–620 (1981)

STEWART D.R., COLODNY A.L. and DAGGETT W.C. Malrotation in infants and children. A 15 year review. *Surgery*, **79,** 716–720 (1976)

Case 30

Answers

		Score
1.	Methaemoglobinaemia (+2) and atrial septal defect (+2).	(+4)
2.	Echocardiogram (+2), give methylene blue (+2); inspect fresh blood sample for chocolate brown appearance (+1), serum methaemoglobin level (+1).	(+4) (+2)
		(+10)

(Average)

Discussion

This boy has central cyanosis. Clinically he also has signs of an atrial septal defect (ASD). A simple ASD however, does not result in cyanosis. His general well being, absence of cardiac failure and normal chest X-ray argue against a significant left to right shunt at atrial level. Despite 'marked cyanosis' this boy's exercise tolerance was reasonable, he did not have digital clubbing and was not polycythaemic. This brings the reliability of the cyanosis due to hypoxia into doubt. Was his blue colour due to some other case? Indeed, a slatey blue-grey discoloration is seen in patients with methaemoglobinaemia who are otherwise generally well. In normal individuals the iron in haemoglobin is maintained in a reduced form by a series of enzymes including cytochrome reductase. Patients with the autosomal recessive form of methaemoglobinaemia have an increased percentage of Fe^{3+} in their haemoglobin due to a defect in the reductase enzyme. This is usually not sufficient to significantly impair their oxygen carrying capacity, but is enough to impart a dark colour to the red cells. Ascorbic acid and methylene blue will reduce the iron to Fe^{2+}, thereby reverting the patient to a normal colour.

Further reading

Methaemoglobinaemia. In *Nelson Textbook of Pediatrics*, 14th edn, Behrman R.E. (ed). W.B. Saunders, Philadelphia, pp. 389–390 (1992)

Methaemoglobinaemia. In *Forfar and Arneil's Textbook of Paediatrics*, 4th edn, Campbell A.G.M., McIntosh N. (eds). Churchill Livingstone, London, pp. 935 (1992)

Methaemoglobinopathies. In *The Metabolic Basis for Inherited Disease*, 6th edn, Scriver C.R., Beaudet A.L., Sly W.S., Valle D. (eds). McGraw Hill, New York, pp. 2267–2280 (1989)

The haemoglobinopathies. In *The Metabolic Basis for Inherited Disease*, 6th edn, Scriver C.R., Beaudet A.L., Sly W.S., Valle D. (eds). McGraw Hill, New York, pp. 2281–2339 (1989)

Case 31

Answers

Score

1. The blood pressure (+0.5), skin rashes (+0.5),
   peripheral pulses (+0.5), eye examination (+0.5). (+2)
2. Anti-nuclear antibodies (ANA, anti-ds antibodies,
   anti-ss antibodies) (+1), anticytoplasmic antibodies
   (ANCA) (+1), renal biopsy (+1); (+3)
   creatinine (+0.5), complement C_3 and C_4 (+0.5),
   ECHO (+0.5). (+1.5)
3. Aseptic bone necrosis. (+1.5)
4. Systemic lupus erythematosis (SLE) or Wegener's
   granulomatosis (WG). (+2)

   ———
   (+10)

Others
Q2: ECG (+0.25).

(Hard)

Discussion

This case history was rather complicated. It may be summarized as follows:

History
8 year old black girl
Prolonged lethargy, aches and pains
Recurrent nasal discharge, chest infections

Examination
Pyrexia
Weight loss
Nasal discharge, large tonsils and soft tissues in upper airways
Hepatosplenomegaly, no lymphadenopathy

Investigation
Bone 'hot spot' with raised ESR but negative cultures
Non-haemolytic anaemia

Relative lymphopenia and thrombocytopenia
Haematuria, proteinuria

This combination of symptoms and signs may be consistent with infection (especially with EBV, HIV or TB), sickle cell disease, a malignancy (especially non-Hodgkin's lymphoma) and connective tissue disease (especially SLE, polyarteritis and Wegener's granulomatosis). The history was rather atypical for infectious mononucleosis and the HIV status and Mantoux were normal. Significant splenomegaly would be unusual in a girl with sickle cell disease at this age. The length of the history and its fluctuating nature argue against lymphoma – besides, bony metastases are unlikely to resolve without intensive chemotherapy! Connective tissue disease (CTD) is generally more common in black people and usually occurs in girls. The vasculitic process involved in these diseases may affect almost any organ and system of the body. Generalized manifestations include fevers, lethargy, aches and weight loss. Skin rashes, polyserositis with effusions and pericarditis, lymphadenopathy, hepatosplenomegaly, anaemia and thrombocytopenia are common features. Involvement of the upper and lower airways is characteristic of Wegener's granulomatosis and results in chronic inflammation and discharge. Bone infarction is not uncommon and renal disease (lupus nephritis in SLE, and a focal necrotising glomerulonephritis in WG) may present with sterile pyuria, proteinuria and microscopic haematuria. Renal involvement may be severe, resulting in renal failure and hypertension. Treatment is based on immunosuppression with steroids, and in refractory cases cyclophosphamide and azathioprime can be used.

Further reading

Systemic lupus erythematosis and Wegener's granulomatosis. In *Nelson Textbook of Pediatrics*, 14th edn, Behrman R.E. (ed). W.B. Saunders, Philadelphia, pp. 624–631 (1992)

Systemic lupus erythematosis and Wegener's granulomatosis. In *Forfar and Arneil's Textbook of Paediatrics*, 4th edn, Campbell A.G.M., McIntosh N. (eds). Churchill Livingstone, London, pp. 1679–1685 (1992)

FISH A.J., BLAU E.B., WESTBERG N.G., BERKE B.A., BERNIER R.G. and MICHAEL A.F. Systemic lupus erythematosis in the first two decades of life. *American Journal of Medicine*, **62**, 99–117 (1977)

KAUFMAN D.B., LAXER R.M., SILVERMAN E.D. and STEIN L. Systemic lupus erythematosis in childhood and adolescence – the problem, epidemiology, incidence, susceptibility, genetics and prognosis. *Current problems in Paediatrics*, **10**, 555–624 (1986)

LEHMAN T.J.A., MCCURDY D.K., BERNSTEIN B.H., KING K.K. and HANSEN V. Systemic lupus erythematosis in the first decade of life. *Pediatrics*, **83**, 235–239 (1989)

HALL S.L., MILLER L.C., DUGGAN E., MAUER S.M., BEATTY E.C. and HELLERSTEIN S. Wegener's granulomatosis in paediatric patients. *Journal of Pediatrics,* **106,** 739–744 (1985)

ORLOWSKI J.H., CLOUGH J.D. and DYMENT P.G. Wegener's granulomatosis in the paediatric age group. *Pediatrics,* **61,** 83–90 (1978)

Case 32

Answers

		Scores
1.	Echocardiogram.	(+2)
2.	Analgesics (+1), diuretics (+1), transfer to paediatric cardiac unit (+2).	(+4)
3.	Fistula from coronary sinus of Valsalva to right atrium.	(+4)

(+10)

Others

Q3: Pericarditis (+1).
Q3: Infective embolus (+0.5), traumatic VSD (+0.5).

(Hard)

Discussion

This girl first presented with partially treated meningitis but made a good recovery and subsequent examination of the CSF was normal. The initial cardiovascular assessment showed no significant abnormality – a soft ejection systolic murmur is not unusual in a sick, pyrexial child with a tachycardia. She re-presented with sudden chest pain followed by breathlessness. Examination on this occasion showed a tachycardia and a significant difference in the systolic and diastolic pressures. This, together with the harsh continuous murmur, would suggest a run-off of blood across a large pressure gradient, and probably from a major artery into a low pressure vessel. Since this girl had also developed pulmonary plethora, it would suggest that there was excess blood flow returning to the right side of the heart. The site of the murmur at the base of the heart would point towards an abnormal connection between the aorta and the right atrium or mediastinal veins, explaining the increased flow into the lungs. A fistula from the coronary sinus of Valsalva to the right atrium would account for this scenario. Other abnormal connections resulting in a pressure run off are less likely: the ductus arteriosus does not reopen in this fashion; aortic dissection does not occur in childhood and traumatic VSDs generally occur in adults with ischaemic heart disease.

Further reading

Rupture, coronary sinus of Valsalva. In *Nelson Textbook of Pediatrics*, 14th edn, Behrman R.E. (ed). W.B. Saunders, Philadelphia, pp. 1174 (1992)

Rupture, coronary sinus of Valsalva. In *Forfar and Arneil's Textbook of Paediatrics*, 4th edn, Campbell A.G.M., McIntosh N. (eds). Churchill Livingstone, London, pp. 680 (1992)

Case 33

Answers

		Score
1.	Congenital cytomegalovirus (CMV) infection.	(+2)
2.	Nasopharyngeal and endotracheal secretions for CMV (+1), urine for CMV culture (+1), urine sediment for owl-eye inclusion bodies (+1), serum for detection of early antigen fluorescing foci (DEAFF) (+1).	(+4)
3.	Blood and platelet transfusions (+1), immunoglobulin (+1), ganciclovir (+1), respiratory support (+1).	(+4)
		(+10)

Others

Q1: Congenital rubella (+1.5); toxoplasmosis (+1); herpes simplex (+0.5); HIV infection (+0.5); syphilis (+0.5).

Q2: Serology for rubella (+0.5), toxoplasmosis (+0.5), herpes (+0.25), HIV (+0.25) or syphilis (+0.25).
Q3: Antibiotics (+0.5).

(Easy)

Discussion

| | Infecting organism | | | | | | | |
	CMV	Rubella	Toxo	Syph	HS	HIV	VZ	HBV
Growth retardation	+	+++	+	+	+	+	+	+
Microcephaly	+	+++	−	−	+	+	+	−
Hydrocephaly	+	−	+++	−	−	+	−	−
CNS calcification	+++	+	++	−	+	−	−	−
Mental retardation	++	++	+	+	+	+	+	−
Chorioretinitis	+	++	+++	+/−	−	−	+	−
Cataracts	−	++	+	−	−	−	+	−
Microphthalmia	+/−	++	+++	−	+	−	+	−
Deafness	++	+++	++	+/−	−	−	−	−
Heart disease	−	++	+	−	−	−	−	−
Pneumonitis	+++	++	++	+	+	+	+	−
Osteitis	++	++	−	+	−	−	−	−
Limb deformities	−	−	−	−	−	+	+	−
Lymphadenopathy	+/−	−	+	+	−	+/−	−	−
Hepatosplenomegaly	++	+++	++++	++	+	+	+	+
Jaundice	++	++	++	+	+	+	+	++
Thrombocytopenia	++	++	+/−	−	−	+/−	−	−
Skin rashes	PP	+/−	−	M,B	S,V	+	CS,V	−

CMV = cytomegalovirus, toxo = toxoplasmosis, syph = syphilis, HS = herpes simplex, HIV = human immunodeficiency virus, VZ = varicella zoster, HBV = hepatitis B virus, PP = pinprick purpura, M = maculopapular, B = bullous, S = scars, V = vesicular, CS = cicatricial scars

The spectrum of clinical and investigative abnormalities presented in this case suggested congenital infection as the probable diagnosis. The differential diagnosis can be summed up by the abbreviation TORCHES which includes: toxoplasmosis (T), (others=O), rubella (R), CMV (C), herpes viruses (simplex and zoster), hepatitis B, HIV (H), enteroviruses (E) and syphilis (S). As shown in the above toxoplasmosis, rubella and CMV would be the more likely infecting organisms in this case. The latter is the most common cause of congenital infection in western countries, affecting 0.4–2.5% of live births, though only 10% develop severe CMV inclusion disease (CID). Intracerebral calcification occurs in all three conditions but is less common with rubella and generally diffuse rather than periventricular in distribution in congenital toxoplasmosis. Eye and congenital heart disease are characteristic of rubella and toxoplasmosis. A pin-point rash, thrombocytopenia and celery stick osteitis (with linear metaphyseal radiolucencies and radiodensities) are common in both congenital CMV and rubella infection.

Further reading

Congenital cytomegalovirus infection. In *Nelson Textbook of Pediatrics*, 14th edn, Behrman R.E. (ed). W.B. Saunders, Philadelphia, pp. 514–515 and 803–805 (1992)

Congenital cytomegalovirus infection. In *Forfar and Arneil's Textbook of Paediatrics*, 4th edn, Campbell A.G.M., McIntosh N. (eds). Churchill Livingstone, London, pp. 314–315; 1420–1421 and 1599 (1992)

YOW M.D. Congenital Cytomegalovirus Disease. A NOW problem. *Journal of Infectious Disease*, **159**, 163–167 (1989)

Case 34

Answers

		Score
1.	Blood culture (+1), joint fluid culture (+1), α-feto-protein level (+1), X-ray knee and chest (+1).	(+4)
2.	Ataxia telangiectasia.	(+2)
3.	Intravenous antibiotics (+1); orthopaedic and physiotherapy involvement (+1); long term physiotherapy and antibiotics for bronchiectasis (+1); genetic counselling (+1).	(+4)
		(+10)

(Average)

Discussion

This boy developed progressive deterioration in his gait and the fact that he is 'clumsy' and falls over suggests that he is now ataxic. He has also had several chest infections and now has evidence of bronchiectasis and possible septic arthritis. The combination of sinopulmonary infection (indicative of IgA deficiency) and ataxia suggests a diagnosis of ataxia telangiectasia. This autosomal recessive disease combines oculocutaneous telangiectases with cerebellar ataxia and variable humoral and cell mediated immunodeficiency. Patients have low or undetectable levels of IgA and IgE. A deficiency in organ maturation is demonstrated by thymic hypoplasia and raised α-feto-protein levels. These patients have a greatly increased sensitivity to irradiation and an increased risk of developing malignant disease. The latter may be the cause of death, though death in early adulthood usually follows progressive bronchiectasis.

Further reading

Ataxia telangiectasia. In *Nelson Textbook of Pediatrics*, 14th edn, Behrman R.E. (ed). W.B. Saunders, Philadelphia, pp. 555–556 (1992)

Ataxia telangiectasia. In *Forfar and Arneil's Textbook of Paediatrics*, 4th edn, Campbell A.G.M., McIntosh N. (eds). Churchill Livingstone, London, pp. 825 and 1314 (1992)

ROSEN F.S., COOPER M.D. and WEDGEWOOD R.J.P. The primary immunodeficiencies. Parts 1 and 2. *New England Journal of Medicine,* **311,** 235 and 300 (1984)

WALDMANN T.A., MISITI J., NELSON D.L. and KRAEMER K.H. Ataxia-telangiectasia: a multisystem hereditary disease with immunodeficiency, impaired organ maturation, X-ray hypersensitivity, and a high incidence of neoplasia. *Annals of Internal Medicine,* **99,** 367–379 (1983)

TAYLOR A.M.R., HARNDEN D.G., ARLETT C.F., HARCOURT S.A., LEHMANN A.R., STEVENS S. and BRIDGES B.A. Ataxia-telangiectasia, a human mutation with abnormal radiation sensitivity. *Nature,* **258,** 427–429 (1975)

Case 35

Answers

		Score
1.	Blood glucose (+0.5), blood gas (+0.5), chest X-ray (+0.5), blood culture (+0.5).	(+2)
2.	Oxygen (+1), intravenous dextrose (+1), antibiotics (+1), physiotherapy (+1), ophthalmological referral (+1).	(+5)
3.	Histamine skin test and methacholine eye test; serum HVA (raised) (+0.5), urine VMA (low) (+0.5).	(+2) (+1)
		(+10)

Others

Q1: Lumbar puncture (+0.25).

(Hard)

Discussion

This girl has global developmental retardation with a tendency toward self-mutilation, severe enough to cause bony fractures and limb deformities. Conditions that involve self-mutilation include Lesch–Nyhan syndrome, congenital sensory neuropathy, leprosy, lead poisoning and familial dysautonomia (Riley–Day syndrome). Children with Riley–Day syndrome present with mental retardation and severe behavioural problems, severe breath holding attacks, recurrent hypoglycaemic episodes, problems with swallowing resulting in recurrent aspiration and chest infections, and an apparent insensitivity to pain. Lack of tears may result in corneal abrasions and repeated trauma and fractures can produce significant chronic deformities. Other manifestations of this recessive condition include poor temperature control, poor taste sensation with lack of fungiform papillae on the tongue, excessive sweating and skin blotching, slurred speech, incoordinate gait and absent tendon reflexes. Autonomic crises may arise in early childhood and manifest as severe cyclical vomiting with hypertension, excessive sweating and skin blotching. Histologically there is a deficiency in unmyelinated fibres supplying the autonomic nervous system and those responsible for peripheral pain and temperature sensation.

Further reading

Riley–Day syndrome. In *Nelson Textbook of Pediatrics*, 14th edn, Behrman R.E. (ed). W.B. Saunders, Philadelphia, pp. 1557–1558 (1992)

Riley–Day syndrome. In *Forfar and Arneil's Textbook of Paediatrics*, 4th edn, Campbell A.G.M., McIntosh N. (eds). Churchill Livingstone, London, pp. 862 and 1180 (1992)

AXELROD F.B., NACHTIGAL R. and DANCIS J. Familial dysautonomia: diagnosis, pathogenesis and management. *Advances in Pediatrics*, **21**, 75–96 (1974)

Case 36

Answers

		Score
1.	HIV status,	(+1)
	Mantoux test (+0.5), early morning urines (+0.5), gastric washings (+0.5), sputum culture (+0.5), T-cell subsets (+0.5), T_4:T_8 ratio (+0.5).	(+3)
2.	Cryptosporidium.	(+1)
3.	Zidovudine (AZT);	(+1)
	antibiotics (+0.5), physiotherapy (+0.5), anti-TB agents (+0.5);	(+1.5)
	potassium supplements (+0.5), calorie additives and TPN (+0.5);	(+1)
	social support (child, mother, addiction and AIDS social services, symptom care/support workers for terminally ill children).	(+1.5)
		(+10)

Others

Q3: Spiromycin (+0.25), imodium (+0.25).

(Average)

Discussion

This child has a chronic illness characterized by marked weight loss, chronic cough and severe diarrhoea. In addition she has anaemia, warts and a pneumonia. This implies that she has some form of immunodeficiency as there are infections at multiple sites. Investigation shows a lymphopenia and since the majority of circulating lymphocytes are of T-cell origin, this suggests a T-cell deficiency. This would fit the picture of a child infected with HIV. The family's social background and mother's generally poor health raise the possibility that the parents themselves may have been intravenous drug abusers. This immediately raises concern regarding infection with HIV. Indeed, not only were all family members HIV positive, but both the mother and child were suffering with AIDS. Patients with AIDS frequently develop chest infections, usually with common organisms, though infections with tuberculosis, *Pneumocystis carinii* and cytomegalovirus are certainly possible. Epstein-Barr virus may be associated with lymphoid interstitial pneumonitis (LIP). Intractable, profuse, offensive diarrhoea may signify gastrointestinal infection with cryptosporidium, and may prove impossible to eradicate. In the active disease the T-helper and T-suppressor (T_4:T_8) cell ratio is reversed (normal range between 1.5–2.3), and hypergammaglobulinaemia (but with impaired function), lymphopenia and thrombocytopenia may develop. Treatment includes the anti-HIV agent zidovudine (AZT), and supportive care – in this case antibiotics and anti-tuberculous drugs, physiotherapy, anti-diarrhoeal agents and improvement in the calorific intake. The latter may necessitate parenteral nutrition and require the insertion of a long-term central line. Finally the social aspects and mother's health cannot be ignored, and social services, the local drug abuse welfare team, adult chest physicians and HIV specialists will all need to be involved in this case.

Further reading

Human immunodeficiency syndrome. In *Nelson Textbook of Pediatrics*, 14th edn, Behrman R.E. (ed). W.B. Saunders, Philadelphia, pp. 835–842 (1992)

Human immunodeficiency syndrome. In *Forfar and Arneil's Textbook of Paediatrics*, 4th edn, Campbell A.G.M., McIntosh N. (eds). Churchill Livingstone, London, pp. 1322–1324, 1451–1457 and 1598–1599 (1992)

BLANCHE S., CANIGLIA M., FISCHER A. *et al*. Zidovudine therapy in children with acquired immunodeficiency syndrome. *American Journal of Medicine*, **85**, 203–207 (1988)

PIZZO P.A., EDDY J. and FALLOON J. Effect of continuous intravenous infusion of zidovudine (AZT) in children with symptomatic HIV infection. *New England Journal of Medicine*, **319**, 889–901 (1985)

FALLOON J., EDDY J., WIENER L. and PIZZO P.A. Human immunodeficiency virus infection in children. *Journal of Pediatrics*, **114**, 1–30 (1989)

Case 37

Answers

		Score
1.	Biopsy bone lesion.	(+2)
2.	Non-malignant proliferation of Langerhans cell histiocytes.	(+2)
3.	Symptomatic support for most cases (+1); steroids (local, and/or systemically) (+1); vinblastine (+1) with or without etoposide (VP16) (+1) in severe disease.	(+4)
4.	The majority remit, sometimes after a chronic relapsing course.	(+2)

(+10)

(Average)

Discussion

Radiolucencies on radiological examination are unusual in pae-diatric practise. They may be due to local bone infection, bone tumours (primary or secondary), benign bony anomalies such as cysts, chondromata and vascular abnormalities. Infection and tumours rarely produce discrete, 'punched out' lesions and the length of the history argues against these possibilities. Congenital anomalies of bone do not generally resolve spontaneously. Recurrent lytic lesions which remit spontaneously are characteristic of Langerhans cell histiocytosis (LCH). This term applies to a spectrum of disease characterized by a non-malignant proliferation of histiocytes. Electron microscopy shows typical tennis racquet shaped Birbeck granules in these cells. The disease may manifest as a solitary lesion in the bone, an eosinophilic granuloma, or may be widely disseminated. The triad of bony lesions, diabetes insipidus (due to CNS involvement) and exophthalmos (due to orbital deposits) is characteristic of Hand–Schuller–Christian disease. The more aggressive Letterer–Siwe disease presents in early childhood with a severe seborrhoeic truncal and perineal rash, lymphadeno-pathy, hepatosplenomegaly and bone marrow infiltration. However, since many children present with features of all three 'syndromes', this classification is no longer in use and all are classified as LCH.

Widespread organ involvement, particularly with organ dysfunction is rare and associated with a poor prognosis. Chronic, intermittently relapsing LCH is more common. Though the disease will eventually remit completely and spontaneously in most patients, some are left with chronic deformities and disabilities. The latter include bony deformities, scoliosis, growth stunting, diabetes insipidus, chronic lung fibrosis, dystrophic nails, dental problems and chronic otitis media. Except for severe widespread disease, treatment is supportive occasionally supplemented with local steroid injections for solitary bony lesions. In those with progressive disease chemotherapy including vinblastine and etoposide have been used with some success.

Further reading

The histiocytoses. In *Nelson Textbook of Pediatrics*, 14th edn, Behrman R.E. (ed). W.B. Saunders, Philadelphia, pp. 1765–1767 (1992)

The histiocytoses. In *Forfar and Arneil's Textbook of Paediatrics*, 4th edn, Campbell A.G.M., McIntosh N. (eds). Churchill Livingstone, London, pp. 1001–1003 (1992)

Writing Up Group of the Histiocyte Society. Histiocytosis syndromes in childhood. *Lancet*, i, 208–209 (1987)

BROADBENT V. Favourable prognostic features in histiocytosis X. *Archives of Disease in Childhood*, 61, 1219–1221 (1986)

Case 38

Answers

		Score
1.	A raised blood pressure or toxic encephalopathy.	(+1)
2	Blood film (+1), clotting screen and FDPs (+1), urinalysis (+1), blood culture (+1), stool culture (*E. coli* with verotoxin) (+1), viral assay (echo, coxsackie, flu) (+1).	(+6)
3.	Peritoneal dialysis (+1), treat hypertension (+1);	(+2)
	transfuse slowly (+0.5), antibiotics (+0.5).	(+1)
		(+10)

116

Q3: Heparin (+0.25), dipyridamole (+0.25), prostacyclin (+0.25).

(Easy)

Discussion

This illness followed a cold and an episode of diarrhoea. The investigations show evidence of haemolysis (severe anaemia and a raised bilirubin) and acute renal failure (uraemia, hyperkalaemia, raised creatinine and acidosis). Therefore, the diagnosis of haemolytic uraemic syndrome (HUS) must be considered. HUS is the commonest cause of acute renal failure in the UK. It usually follows a bacterial or viral infection of the gut or upper airways in young children, often in the summer months. Sporadic cases do occur, often in older children where the outcome is generally worse. Hypertension is a common complication of this condition and, as in this case, may result in a hypertensive encephalopathy with convulsions. Fluid retention secondary to the oliguria or anuria and the hypertension account for the cardiac failure.

In this condition endothelial cell injury, particularly in the kidneys, is associated with a mechanical microangiopathic haemolytic process and platelet consumption. Haematological investigations show burr and fragmented red cells, schistocytes, a Coombs' negative anaemia, thrombocytopenia and a leucocytosis. Frank disseminated intravascular coagulation is uncommon. Urinalysis shows haematuria and proteinuria and biochemical tests confirm the acute renal failure. The management includes correction of the anaemia and the uraemia preferably with early peritoneal dialysis. Strict control of the fluid balance and hypertension is essential, and secondary infections should be prevented. Heparin and anti-platelet agents have been employed in the acute phase with variable results. The majority of patients will survive the acute illness and regain normal renal function.

Further reading

Haemolytic uraemic syndrome. In *Nelson Textbook of Pediatrics*, 14th edn, Behrman R.E. (ed). W.B. Saunders, Philadelphia, pp. 1334–1336 (1992)

Haemolytic uraemic syndrome. In *Forfar and Arneil's Textbook of Paediatrics*, 4th edn, Campbell A.G.M., McIntosh N. (eds). Churchill Livingstone, London, pp. 1064–1066 (1992)

SIEGLER R.L.. Management of haemolytic uraemic syndrome. *Journal of Pediatrics,* **112,** 1014–1020 (1988)

SIEGLER R.L., MILLIGAN M.R., BURNINGHAM T.H. *et al.* Long-term outcome and prognostic indications in the haemolytic uraemic syndrome. *Journal of Pediatrics,* **118,** 195–200 (1991)

NOVILLO A.A., VOYER L.E., CRAVIOTO R. Haemolytic uraemic syndrome associated with faecal cytotoxin and verotoxin neutralising antibodies. *Pediatric Nephrology,* **1,** 566–573 (1988)

SCHLIEPER A., ROWE P.C., ORRBINE E. *et al.* Sequelae of haemolytic uraemic syndrome. *Archives of Disease in Childhood,* **67,** 930–934 (1992)

Case 39

Answers

		Score
1.	Hypoproteinaemia (+0.5), vitamin D (+0.5) and vit. K deficiency (+0.5), folate deficiency (+0.5).	(+2)
2.	Jejunal biopsy;	(+1)
	albumin (+0.5), serum folate (+0.5), X-ray wrist and ankles (+0.5), 24 hour stool fat content (+0.5), assess gastrointestinal protein loss using Cr^{51} labelled albumin (+0.5).	(+2.5)
3.	Intestinal lymphangiectasia.	(+2.5)
4.	High protein diet (+0.5), medium chain triglycerides (MCT) (+0.5), fat soluble vitamin (+0.5) and folate supplements (+0.5).	(+2)
		(+10)

Others

Q1: Vitamin B_{12} deficiency (+0.25).
Q3: Whipple's disease (+1.5), intestinal lymphoma (+1).

(Hard)

Discussion

This patient has developed malabsorption. The metabolic problems are explained by the malabsorption of fat and fat soluble vitamins. In addition he has a megaloblastic anaemia which, in view

118

of the short history, is more likely to be due to folate deficiency rather than vitamin B_{12} deficiency. However, there is increased loss of protein in the stools (i.e. elevated α_1-antitrypsin excretion) and, therefore, he also has a protein losing enteropathy. This combination of malabsorption with protein losing enteropathy is seen with intestinal lymphoma, Whipple's disease, intestinal lymphangiectasia, inflammatory bowel disease (IBD) and cystic fibrosis. The normal contrast study makes IBD unlikely; the normal sweat test excludes cystic fibrosis and the normal abdominal ultrasound mitigates against a lymphoma. Whipple's disease is usually associated with arthralgia and fevers, but not with pedal oedema and a lymphopenia. Though the latter is suggestive of intestinal lymphangiectasia, the diagnosis can only be confirmed by a jejunal biopsy.

Further reading

Intestinal lymphangiectasia. In *Nelson Textbook of Pediatrics*, 14th edn, Behrman R.E. (ed). W.B. Saunders, Philadelphia, pp. 982 (1992)

Intestinal lymphangiectasia. In *Forfar and Arneil's Textbook of Paediatrics*, 4th edn, Campbell A.G.M., McIntosh N. (eds). Churchill Livingstone, London, pp. 512–513 (1992)

STROBER W., WOCHNER R.D., CARBONE P.P. and WALDMANN T.A. Intestinal lymphangiectasia. A protein losing enteropathy with hypogammaglobulinaemia, lymphocytopenia and impaired homograft rejection. *Journal of Clinical Investigation*, **46**, 1643–1656 (1967)

VARDY P.A., LEBENTHAL E. and SHWACHMAN H. Intestinal lymphangiectasia: a reappraisal. *Journal of Pediatrics*, **55**, 842–851 (1975)

WALDMANN T.A. Protein losing enteropathy. *Gastroenterology*, **50**, 422–443 (1966)

Lymphangiectasia. In *Diseases of the Small Intestine in Childhood*, 3rd edn, Walker-Smith J.A. (ed). Butterworth, London, pp. 421–425 (1988)

Lymphangiectasia. In *Pediatric Gastrointestinal Disease*, Walker W.A., Durie P.R., Amilton J.R., Walker-Smith J.A., Watkin J.B. (eds). B.C. Becker, pp. 814–815 (1991)

Case 40

Answers

		Score
1.	Henoch-Schönlein (anaphylactoid) purpura.	(+4)
2.	Admit and observe (+3); analgesics (+3).	(+6)
		————
		(+10)
		(Easy)

Discussion

The description of the rash and its distribution in a child who is generally well is consistent with a vasculitic rash seen in Henoch-Schönlein (anaphylactoid) purpura (HSP). HSP is a benign, self-limiting condition which generally resolves, sometimes after a short fluctuating course. Almost 50% of affected children have gastrointestinal symptoms including colicky pains and frank or occult blood in the stool. Only rarely are these symptoms associated with an intussusception, perforation or bowel obstruction. A transient, flitting non-deforming arthropathy is a common feature of this condition, arising in approximately 60% of cases. Renal involvement occurs in 25–50% of cases, and is usually limited to haematuria. The development of chronic renal disease is extremely rare and may result in hypertension, nephrotic syndrome and nephritis. Scrotal, testicular and neurological complications have also been described. A combination of a vasculitic rash, haematuria and abdominal pain can also be seen with lupus disease, polyarteritis and Goodpastures syndrome – but in these conditions the patient is usually acutely unwell.

Further reading

Henoch–Schönlein purpura. In *Nelson Textbook of Pediatrics*, 14th edn, Behrman R.E. (ed). W.B. Saunders, Philadelphia, pp. 628–629 (1992)

Henoch–Schönlein purpura. In *Forfar and Arneil's Textbook of Paediatrics*, 4th edn, Campbell A.G.M., McIntosh N. (eds). Churchill Livingstone, London, pp. 947 and 1683–1685 (1992)

ALLEN D.M., DIAMOND L.K. and HOWELL D.A. Anaphylactoid purpura in children (Henoch-Schönlein Syndrome). Review with follow up of renal complications. *American Journal of Disease in Childhood*, **99**, 833–854 (1960)

Case 41

Answers

		Score
1.	Nephroblastoma (Wilms' tumour) extending into the inferior vena cava and right atrium.	(+2)
2.	Tricuspid regurgitation secondary to tumour disrupting function of tricuspid valve.	(+2)
3.	Echocardiogram.	(+2)
4.	Treat heart failure (+1), chemotherapy (+1);	(+2)
	surgery (combined cardiac and renal).	(+2)

$$(+10)$$

Others

Q1: Nephroblastoma (Wilms' tumour) (+1).

(Hard)

Discussion

The initial presentation with a large right-sided abdominal mass and haematuria was indicative of nephroblastoma. Of note were the ultrasound findings – a right-sided mass presumably obliterating the right kidney and right adrenal gland (not an uncommon state of affairs with large Wilms' tumours), but also obscuring the IVC. The latter raised the possibility of IVC invasion with tumour, a rare but well described complication of right-sided Wilms' tumours. The patient then went on to develop signs consistent with tricuspid incompetence. The explanation for this new finding was disruption of the tricuspid valve due to tumour-thrombus impinging onto the valve. The real-time echocardiographic images of similar tumours 'ball valving' through the tricuspid valve and impeding its closure are, needless to say, rather dramatic! The management of choice is combined cardio-renal surgery to remove the tumour en bloc. However, this child is in congestive cardiac failure and this needs to be addressed preoperatively. It is also standard practise to give the first dose of chemotherapy prior to surgery for nephroblastoma in order to minimize the risk of metastatic spread.

Further reading

Wilms' tumour. In *Nelson Textbook of Pediatrics*, 14th edn, Behrman R.E. (ed). W.B.
Saunders, Philadelphia, pp. 1307–1309 (1992)

Wilms' tumour. In *Forfar and Arneil's Textbook of Paediatrics*, 4th edn, Campbell
A.G.M., McIntosh N. (eds). Churchill Livingstone, London, pp. 987–989 (1992)

D'ANGIO G.J., EVANS A.E., BRESLOW N. *et al*. The treatment of Wilms' tumor. Results of the
Second National Wilms' Tumor Study. *Cancer*, **47**, 2302–2311 (1981)

Oncological emergencies: intracardiac tamponade. In *Principles and Practise of
Pediatric Oncology*, 2nd edn, Pizzo P.A., Poplack D.G. (eds). J.B. Lippincott,
Philadelphia, pp. 954 (1993)

Case 42

Answers

		Score
1.	Sweat test by iontophoresis at 6 weeks of age;	(+1.5)
	immunoreactive trypsin.	(+1.5)
2.	Regular physiotherapy (+1), antibiotics (+1), stoma care (+1), optimize calorific intake (±TPN) (+1), pancreatic supplements (+1), vitamin E supplements (+1), genetic counselling (+1).	(+7)
		(+10)

Others

Q1: Stool trypsin activity (+0.5).

(Easy)

Discussion

The combination of bowel obstruction and respiratory problems in the neonatal period is suggestive of cystic fibrosis. The clinical, radiological and laparotomy findings were consistent with a diagnosis of meconium ileus. Furthermore, this child's post-operative course was complicated by pulmonary consolidation and collapse due to viscid pulmonary secretions.

In the UK, 1 in 25 are carriers for this autosomal recessive condition and 1 in 2500 children will suffer from the disease.

Furthermore, 5 out of every 6 patients with meconium ileus have cystic fibrosis. In this condition the bowel is full of plugs and columns of tacky inspissated meconium, and may remain partly under-developed. The treatment involves a defunctioning ileostomy with a clearout of meconium plugs, followed by re-anastomosis at a later date. Management of the respiratory problem includes regular physiotherapy, regular courses of antibiotics and prophylactic antibiotics initially against *Staphylococcus aureus* and *Haemophilus influenzae. Pseudomonas aeruginosa* is a problem in later child-hood. Frequent high lipase pancreatic supplements vitamin E and increased calories are essential dietary measures. Screening for the abnormal gene on chromosome 7 is possible in 90% of families and gene therapy is currently under review as part of the treatment for the respiratory tract.

Further reading

Cystic fibrosis. In *Nelson Textbook of Pediatrics*, 14th edn, Behrman R.E. (ed). W.B. Saunders, Philadelphia, pp. 1106–1116 (1992)

Cystic fibrosis. In *Forfar and Arneil's Textbook of Paediatrics*, 4th edn, Campbell A.G.M., McIntosh N. (eds). Churchill Livingstone, London, pp. 518–520, 557–558 and 625–633 (1992)

GASKIN K.J., WATERS D.L.M., HOWMAN-GILES R.N. *et al.* Liver disease and common bile duct stenosis in cystic fibrosis. *New England Journal of Medicine,* **318**, 340–346 (1988)

PARK R., GRAND R.J. Gastrointestinal manifestations of cystic fibrosis. *Gastroenterology,* **81**, 1143–1161 (1981)

BUCHDAHL R.M., FULLEYLOVE C., MARCHANT J.L. *et al.* Energy and nutrient intake in cystic fibrosis. *Archives of Disease in Childhood,* **64**, 373–378 (1989)

DORATI M.A., GUENETTE G. and AUERBACH H. Prospective controlled study of home and hospital therapy and cystic fibrosis pulmonary disease. *Journal of Pediatrics,* **111**, 28–33 (1987)

COUTELLE C., CALPEN N., HART S. *et al.* Gene therapy for cystic fibrosis. *Archives of Disease in Childhood,* **68**, 437–440 (1993)

STUART ELBORN J. Cystic fibrosis: prospects for gene therapy. *Hospital Update,* **20**, 13–22 (1994)

Case 43

Answers

		Score
1.	Osteomyelitis or septic arthritis.	(+2)
2.	Incorrect route and choice of antibiotic.	(+2)
3.	X-ray left arm (+1); bone scan (+1); repeated blood cultures (+1); orthopaedic assessment (+1); intravenous penicillin for 10–14 days followed by oral penicillin for 4 weeks (+2).	(+6)

(+10)

(Easy)

Discussion

This baby presented with a septicaemic episode due to a β-haemo-lytic streptococcus. The correct treatment in this situation is penicillin G given intravenously for 10–14 days, followed by penicillin V for at least 4 weeks. Therefore, in this case, both the choice of antibiotic regimen and route of administration are inappropriate. On re-admission the patient was pyrexial and had developed a pseudoparalysis of the left upper limb. Pseudoparaly-sis in this age group is usually due to birth trauma or infection. In this case, following the preceding septicaemia, a secondary osteomyel-itis/septic arthritis had developed. Bony changes may be evident on an X-ray at this stage (and in fact showed a lytic area in the upper humeral metaphysis). A bone scan would show an area of increased tracer uptake in the affected area. Management includes antibiotics and surgical drainage for a septic arthritis and for osteomyelitis that does not improve with antibiotics alone.

Further reading

Neonatal sepsis. In *Nelson Textbook of Pediatrics*, 14th edn, Behrman R.E. (ed). W.B. Saunders, Philadelphia, pp. 501–504 (1992)

Osteomyelitis. In *Nelson Textbook of Pediatrics*, 14th edn, Behrman R.E. (ed). W.B. Saunders, Philadelphia, pp. 691–694 (1992)

Osteomyelitis. In *Forfar and Arneil's Textbook of Paediatrics*, 4th edn, Campbell A.G.M., McIntosh N. (eds). Churchill Livingstone, London, pp. 310–311 and 1662–1664 (1992)

Case 44

Answers

Score

1. Blood glucose (+2), urine glucose (+2), urine
ketones (+2). (+6)
2. Insulin-dependent diabetic ketoacidosis. (+4)

(+10)

Others

Q1: Urine osmolality (+1).

(Average)

Discussion

The chance of a relapse 7 years after completion of treatment for Hodgkin's disease is extremely small. Hence, this illness was unlikely to be related to the previous malignant disease. This boy presented with a short history of vomiting and a deteriorating conscious level. Investigations showed evidence of dehydration (raised haematocrit and urea) and a hyperosmolar state, not accounted for by any of the electrolyte results provided in the case report. The most likely cause for the hyperosmolality would be a raised serum glucose level, making acute diabetic ketoacidosis the most likely diagnosis. Indeed, up to 25% of children with IDDM may first present with ketoacidosis.

Further reading

Diabetic ketoacidosis. In *Nelson Textbook of Pediatrics*, 14th edn, Behrman R.E. (ed). W.B. Saunders, Philadelphia, pp. 390–408 (1992)

Diabetic ketoacidosis. In *Forfar and Arneil's Textbook of Paediatrics*, 4th edn, Campbell A.G.M., McIntosh N. (eds). Churchill Livingstone, London, pp. 1146–1154 (1992)

FOSTER D.W. and MCGARRY J.D. The metabolic derangement and treatment of diabetic ketoacidosis. *New England Journal of Medicine*, **309**, 159–169 (1983)

HARRIS G.D., FIORDALINI I. and FINBERG I. Safe management of diabetic ketoacidosis. *Journal of Pediatrics*, **113**, 65–68 (1988)

KRANE E.J., ROCKOFF M.A., WALLMAN J.K. and WOLFSDORF J.I. Subclinical brain swelling in children during treatment of diabetic ketoacidosis. *New England Journal of Medicine*, **312**, 1147–1151 (1985)

ROSENBLOOM A.L., RILEY W.J., WEBER F.T. *et al.* Cerebral oedema complicating diabetic ketoacidosis in children. *Journal of Pediatrics,* **96,** 357–361 (1980)

JOHNSTON D.I. Management of diabetes mellitus. *Archives of Disease in Childhood,* **64,** 622–628 (1989)

Case 45

Answers

		Score
1.	Examine eyes (+1), genitals (+1), attempt to pass nasogastric tube through both nostrils (+1).	(+3)
2.	Eye and ENT examination (EUA) (+1), auditory evoked responses (+1), echocardiogram (+1), abdominal ultrasound (+1).	(+4)
3.	CHARGE associated with choanal atresia, a ventricular septal defect (VSD) and ear abnormality.	(+3)
		———
		(+10)
		(Average)

Discussion

Once intubated, this baby required minimal artificial support in order to maintain adequate ventilation. However, when allowed to breathe spontaneously he rapidly developed marked recession and respiratory distress. This history suggests that the gas exchange at alveolar level was normal, and the problem was overcome by oral intubation or improved with mouth opening (crying). Therefore, there is a problem in the upper nasal airways, and one explanation which would account for this would be choanal atresia (A). Up to 50% of children with choanal atresia have other congenital abnormalities. Indeed, this child had a vestigial ear (E) and a congenital heart defect (H), probably a ventricular septal defect. These anomalies are found together with colobomas (C), retardation (R) and genital anomalies (G) in the CHARGE association.

Further reading

CHARGE syndrome. In *Nelson Textbook of Pediatrics*, 14th edn, Behrman R.E. (ed). W.B. Saunders, Philadelphia, pp. 1053 (1992)

CHARGE association. In *Smith's Recognizable Patterns of Human Malformation*, 4th edn, Jones K.L. (ed). W.B. Saunders, Philadelphia, pp. 606–608 (1988)

HALL B.D. Choanal atresia and associated multiple anomalies. *Journal of Pediatrics*, **95**, 395–398 (1979)

BLAKE K., KIRK J.M.W. and UR E. Growth in CHARGE association. *Archives of Disease in Childhood*, **68**, 508–509 (1993)

Case 46

Answers

		Score
1.	Steady progression in height and weight below but parallel to the 3rd centile;	(+2)
	improvement in social skills after the foster placement.	(+2)
2.	Russel Silver dwarfism.	(+3)
3.	Maintain foster placement.	(+3)
		(+10)

Others

Q2: Fetal alcohol syndrome (+1).

(Average)

Discussion

The causes of failure to thrive are legion and can include problems in almost every system in the body. In the context of this case presentation, the main possibilities would include: emotional deprivation and social neglect; intra-uterine problems including fetal alcohol syndrome and idiopathic intra-uterine growth retardation (IUGR); hypothyroidism, growth hormone deficiency and various syndromes. Social and emotional neglect could be a possibility though this child was uniformly small at birth and had a normal growth velocity, below but parallel to the 3rd centile line. There was no improvement in linear growth when she was placed with foster parents, though her social skills had improved. There is little evidence for IUGR and hypothyroidism is virtually ruled out by the normal T_4 result. Fetal alcohol syndrome generally results in a small child who may continue to grow poorly after birth and may well be developmentally delayed. However, the physical description of this child with pixie-like petite features (due to frontal bossing and a small triangular face), particularly small hands (usually with clinodactly), and dwarf-like proportions was in keeping with a diagnosis of Russel-Silver dwarfism. These children grow along a line well below the 3rd centile and have mild to moderate development delay. Hemi-hypertrophy and café au lait spots are also associated with this condition. These children have a surge in growth hormone after a provocation test. While they may show an initial response to growth hormone therapy, this is not always sustained in the long term. In this case, in view of the improvement in social skills, it would be appropriate to leave the child with foster parents.

Further reading

Russel–Silver syndrome. In *Nelson Textbook of Pediatrics*, 14th edn, Behrman R.E. (ed). W.B. Saunders, Philadelphia, pp. 1402 (1992)

Russel–Silver syndrome. In *Forfar and Arneil's Textbook of Paediatrics*, 4th edn, Campbell A.G.M., McIntosh N. (eds). Churchill Livingstone, London, pp. 1103 (1992)

Russel–Silver syndrome. In *Smith's Recognizable Patterns of Human Malformation*, 4th edn, Jones K.L. (ed). W.B. Saunders, Philadelphia, pp. 88–89 (1988)

SILVER H.K. Asymmetry, short stature and variation in sexual development. A syndrome of congenital malformation. *American Journal of Disease in Childhood.* **107,** 495–515 (1964)

Case 47

Answers

Score

1. Betadine induced, temporary hypothyroidism.   (+ 10)

Others

Q1: Goitrogen-induced hypothyroidism (+8).
Q1: Stress induced, transient hypothyroidism (+6).

(Hard)

Discussion

This neonate had unequivocal but transient hypothyroidism. Indeed the thyroid function at the age of 20 weeks, and 12 weeks after discontinuing thyroid hormone replacements, was normal. Additional investigation confirmed the presence of a normally sited gland with normal uptake on an isotope scan, and excluded dyshormonogenesis and antibody-related causes of hypothyroidism. Likewise, the maternal thyroid function was normal and there was no evidence for maternal goitrogens. However, temporary exposure to a goitrogen shortly after birth could not be excluded. This child had a significant gastroschisis at birth and the loops of exposed, oedematous bowel were wrapped in betadine-soaked swabs. It is probable that this mode of treatment resulted in significant absorption of povidone iodine which adversely affected the neonatal thyroid gland, and resulted in transient hypothyroidism. Once the exposure to betadine was discontinued the thyroid function returned to normal.

Further reading

Hypothyroidism. In *Nelson Textbook of Pediatrics*, 14th edn, Behrman R.E. (ed). W.B. Saunders, Philadelphia, pp. 1418 (1992)

COSMAN B.C., SCHULLINGER J.N., BELL J.J., REGAN J.A. Hypothroidism caused by topical povidine-iodine in a newborn with omphalocele. *Journal of Pediatric Surgery*, **23**, 356–358 (1988)

SMITH D.W., KLEIN A.M., HENDERSON J.R. Congenital hypothyroidism – signs and symptoms in the newborn period. *Journal of Pediatrics*, **87**, 958–962 (1975)

MAGEE P. Adverse reactions profile: Povidone-iodine. *Prescriber's Journal*, **33**, 160–163 (1993)

Case 48

Answers

		Score
1.	Sleep or resting EEG studies.	(+4)
2.	Polyspike wave discharges in centrotemporal area typical of benign partial rolandic epilepsy of childhood.	(+3)
3.	Reassurance (+1.5); carbamazepine if convulsion frequency deteriorates (+1.5).	(+3)
		(+10)

Others

Q1: EEG (+3).
Q3: Any other anticonvulsant (+1).

(Average)

Discussion

The history is characteristic of benign rolandic epilepsy of childhood (or benign partial epilepsy with centrotemporal spikes – BPEC). This condition comprises up to 15–20% of childhood epilepsy, arising in healthy children aged 3–13 years with a peak of 9–10 years. The majority of the fits occur during sleep, though some children will experience a seizure first thing in the morning. The episodes are typified by an altered sensation and tonic contractions of the tongue, cheeks and lips followed by slurred speech, grunting, excessive salivation and drooling. Twitching around the mouth is a frequent accompaniment and may progress to tonic-clonic contractions of the lower face. Progression to a generalized fit is also possible with subsequent loss rather than alteration in the conscious level. The EEG is characterized by unilateral or bilateral repetitive, high amplitude, spike discharges in the presylvian (rolandic) or centrotemporal area. The changes on the EEG are far more pronounced during sleep. Most patients will experience less than 5 fits, remain unaware of their seizures which, in the majority of patients, remit spontaneously during puberty. Only those patients with frequent seizures may require anticonvulsants, and carbamazepine is the drug of choice.

Further reading

Benign partial epilepsy. In *Nelson Textbook of Pediatrics*, 14th edn, Behrman R.E. (ed). W.B. Saunders, Philadelphia, pp. 1493–1494 (1992)

Benign partial epilepsy. In *Forfar and Arneil's Textbook of Paediatrics*, 4th edn, Campbell A.G.M., McIntosh N. (eds). Churchill Livingstone, London, pp. 762–763 (1992)

Benign focal epilepsia of childhood. In *Recent Advances in Epilepsy*, Vol. 3, Pedley T.A., Meldrum B.S. (eds). Churchill Livingstone, Edinburgh, pp. 137–156 (1986)

CLEMENS B. and OHAH R. Sleep studies in benign epilepsy of childhood with Rolandic spikes: sleep pathology. *Epilepsia*, **28,** 20–23 (1987)

Case 49

Answers

		Score
1.	Volume replacement (+1), nil by mouth (+1), nasogastric tube and aspirate stomach (+1), correct electrolytes disorders (+1).	(+4)
2.	Full thickness bowel biopsy (+2), intestinal manometry (+2).	(+4)
3.	Chronic intermittent intestinal pseudo-obstruction (CIIP).	(+2)
		(+10)

Others

Q1: Antibiotics (+0.5).
Q2: Creatinine (+1); intravenous pyelogram (+1); mictuating cystourethrogram (+1).

(Hard)

Discussion

This unusual story was consistent with recurrent bowel obstruction. Initial investigation did not show any anatomical bowel abnormality such as a malrotation or congenital anomaly, and there was no evidence of mucosal disease. Following recurrent bouts of bowel stasis and partial obstruction, he underwent a laparotomy at the age of 4 years. Despite an ileus and multiple loops of distended bowel, no mechanical obstruction was found at operation. This suggests that the problem was inherent to the intestine, and more specifically, to an abnormality in intestinal motility. This situation occurs in a few rare heterogenous conditions involving dysfunctional peristalsis, and is grouped under the term chronic intermittent intestinal pseudo-obstruction (CIIP). The condition may be familial and the underlying cause is a visceral myopathy or visceral neuropathy which may be demonstrated on a full thickness bowel biopsy. Intestinal manometry is the most useful investigation, showing low amplitude, disrupted or uncoordinated motor peristaltic pressure waves. Absence of the normal fasting motor activity results in an ileus, intraluminal stasis, bacterial overgrowth with gaseous distention and pseudo-obstruction. Associated urinary problems arise in 30% of patients and include megaureters, megacystis and an increased risk of urinary tract infections. The condition must be differentiated from mechanical obstruction, Hirschsprung's disease and psychogenic vomiting. Narcotic abuse, hypothyroidism, diabetes mellitus and porphyria must also be excluded. Furthermore, any male child with bilateral megaureters must be investigated for posterior urethral valves and renal failure. Treatment is difficult and may involve long-term parenteral nutrition.

Further reading

Chronic intermittent intestinal pseudo-obstruction. In *Nelson Textbook of Pediatrics*, 14th edn, Behrman R.E. (ed). W.B. Saunders, Philadelphia, pp. 960 (1992)

Chronic intermittent intestinal pseudo-obstruction. In *Forfar and Arneil's Textbook of Paediatrics*, 4th edn, Campbell A.G.M., McIntosh N. (eds). Churchill Livingstone, London, pp. 521 (1992)

Case 50

Answers

		Score
1.	Atrioventricular septal defect.	(+2)
2.	Echocardiogram (+1), chest X-ray (+1), repeated blood cultures (+1).	(+3)
3.	Treat cardiac failure (+1); intravenous antibiotics for 6 weeks (+1); blood transfusion (+1).	(+3)
4.	Pulmonary hypertension exacerbated by infection.	(+2)
		(+10)

Others

Q2: ECG (+0.5); repeat cardiac catheterization (+0.5).
Q3: Treat any arrhythmias (+1).
Q4: Arrhythmias (+0.5); dislodged dacron patch (+0.5).

(Hard)

Discussion

The first paragraph of this report summarized this girl's initial problems, namely Down's syndrome with an atrioventricular septal defect (AVSD). The latter is the most common lesion seen in children with trisomy 21. A superior axis on the ECG is seen in tricuspid atresia (TA) and AVSD. The latter, unlike TA, does not result in persistent cyanosis and classically presents with cardiac failure. It is not an aggregation of an ASD plus a VSD, but is a complex defect straddling all four cardiac chambers which are separated in the centre by a single abnormal atrioventricular valve. The latter is morphologically dissimilar to a tricuspid or mitral valve and is almost invariably incompetent. The predominant shunt is from the left ventricle to the right atrium, and thence into the lungs. The increase in pulmonary blood flow may reach torrential proportions and results in heart failure with marked cardiomegaly and pulmonary plethora. As compared to a VSD, the risk of developing pulmonary hypertension is greatly increased. In addition, the time interval before this occurs in children with Down's syndrome is greatly reduced.

This infant was investigated at a late stage and was shown to have a degree of pulmonary hypertension which appeared to be reversible. The corrective operation for AVSD involves closure of the septal defect and, if necessary, repair of the left-sided AV valve leaflet. A degree of AV valve regurgitation is almost inevitable although right-sided regurgitation is well tolerated. Therefore, all such children will have a residual post-operative pansystolic murmer (PSM). Despite the operative repair this baby fared badly and eventually succumbed after progressive cyanosis and heart failure. There are a number of possibilities to account for the post-operative course. Dislodgement of the Dacron patch may have occurred but would have produced acute cardiac embarrassment. While a small residual 'VSD' around the patch could account for the residual murmur and contributed to a degree of cardiac failure due to a left-to-right shunt, it would not have resulted in marked cyanosis. This baby developed a post-operative infection involving the central line and neither a post-operative pneumonia nor bacterial endocarditis can be excluded (especially in view of the artificial Dacron *in situ*). Both these infections would certainly exacerbate any pre-existing pulmonary hypertension. Furthermore, in view of the intermittent 'mottling' in the post-operative period, an arrhythmia is another possible complication.

Further reading

Pulmonary hypertension and cardiac disease. In *Nelson Textbook of Pediatrics*, 14th edn, Behrman R.E. (ed). W.B. Saunders, Philadelphia, pp. 1162–1163 (1992)

Pulmonary hypertension and cardiac disease. In *Forfar and Arneil's Textbook of Paediatrics*, 4th edn, Campbell A.G.M., McIntosh N. (eds). Churchill Livingstone, London, pp. 678–679 (1992)

HOFFMAN J.I.E., RUDOLPH A.M. and HEYMANN M.A. Pulmonary vascular disease with congenital heart lesions. Pathologic features and causes. *Circulation*, **64**, 873–877 (1981)

Case 51

Answers

Score

1. Attach ECG monitor (+2), dextrose infusion (+2),
   anticonvulsant if fits persist (+2).   (+6)
2. Urine/serum samples for drug toxicology.   (+4)

    (+10)

(Easy)

Discussions

This boy presented in an unconscious state with seizures, depression of most neurological responses, hypothermia and relative hypotension. No causative factors could be found on examination and detailed investigation. In children the sudden onset of unexplained neurological signs, particularly if accompanied by abnormal movements, cardiovascular decompensation and hypoglycaemia should raise the suspicion of inappropriate ingestion of drugs or poisons. In this case the social history and the knowledge of this boy's renegade behaviour added weight to this diagnosis. Indeed, following a bet with his brother, he had ingested several haloperidol tablets which he had found in the hospital's refuse collection area!

Further reading

Self poisoning. In *Nelson Textbook of Pediatrics*, 14th edn, Behrman R.E. (ed). W.B. Saunders, Philadelphia, pp. 1775–1782 (1992)

Self poisoning. In *Forfar and Arneil's Textbook of Paediatrics*, 4th edn, Campbell A.G.M., McIntosh N. (eds). Churchill Livingstone, London, pp. 1778–1784 (1992)

ELLISON D.W. and PENTEL P.R. Clinical features and complications of seizures due to cyclic antidepressant overdose. *American Journal of Emergency Medicine*, **7**, 5–10 (1989)

Case 52

Answers

		Score
1.	Haemophilia A (moderate factor VIII deficiency).	(+5)
2.	Turner's syndrome.	(+5)

(+10)

(Easy)

Discussion

There were two aspects to this case. The first was the cause of this child's bruising. The history of easy bruising, joint swelling after minor injury, prolonged PT and KPPT times together with a reduced level of factor VIII all point toward a diagnosis of haemophilia A. However, this is a classical X-linked recessive condition *par excellance*! How, therefore, could this disease manifest in a girl? For a girl to develop haemophilia A, she must be homozygous, having inherited two abnormal X-chromosomes, one from a carrier mother and the other from an affected father. In this case the answer lies in the information provided regarding this girl's short stature and the absence of any signs of pubertal development at the age of 13 years. The latter combination is seen in girls with Turner's syndrome. If the single X-chromosome in a girl with Turner's syndrome carries the recessive gene for haemophilia, then the same situation arises as in boys who develop the disease. These girls will also express the abnormal gene and develop a bleeding tendency.

Further reading

Turner's syndrome. In *Nelson Textbook of Pediatrics*, 14th edn, Behrman R.E. (ed). W.B. Saunders, Philadelphia, pp. 292–293 and 1460–1462 (1992)

Turner's syndrome. In *Forfar and Arneil's Textbook of Paediatrics*, 4th edn, Campbell A.G.M., McIntosh N. (eds). Churchill Livingstone, London, pp. 67–68, 435–437, 1077 and 1093 (1992)

Turner's syndrome. In *Smith's Recognizable Patterns of Human Malformation*, 4th edn, Jones K.L. (ed). W.B. Saunders, Philadelphia, pp. 74–79 (1988)

Haemophilia. In *Nelson Textbook of Pediatrics*, 14th edn, Behrman R.E. (ed). W.B. Saunders, Philadelphia, pp. 1275–1277 (1992)

136

Haemophilia. In *Forfar and Arneil's Textbook of Paediatrics*, 4th edn, Campbell A.G.M., McIntosh N. (eds). Churchill Livingstone, London, pp. 950–952 (1992)

Case 53

Answers

		Score
1.	Fundoscopy (+2), visual fields (+2), pulse and blood pressure (+2).	(+6)
2.	CT brain scan.	(+4)
		(+10)

Others

Q1: Neurological examination (+1).

(Easy)

Discussion

There are many causes of vomiting in childhood. The large majority of cases are not associated with any serious underlying pathology. In this case the vomiting was severe enough to cause an oesophagitis with chronic upper gastrointestinal bleeding and result in an iron deficiency anaemia. Such severe vomiting may be seen in psychosomatic conditions such as cyclical vomiting. However, before a 'non-organic' diagnosis is made in this case, other features associated with the vomiting must first be considered. The vomiting occurred mostly in the mornings and was associated with headaches and drowsiness, all possible features of raised intracranial pressure (ICP). The latter may be a manifestation of pseudotumour cerebri and a space occupying lesion. Bradycardia, hypertension, papilloedema and visual field defects are clinical signs indicative of raised ICP, whereas cranial nerve III, IV and VI palsies are false localizing signs. Nevertheless, a normal neurological examination does not necessarily rule out an intracranial space occupying lesion. In this case further investigation was indicated on the strength of the history alone. A CT brain scan with contrast would be the investigation of choice. In this child, a CT scan confirmed a large tumour in the posterior fossa with obstruction of the fourth ventricle and a degree of hydrocephalus despite a normal examination. Biopsy subsequently confirmed a medulloblastoma.

Further reading

Brain tumours. In *Nelson Textbook of Pediatrics*, 14th edn, Behrman R.E. (ed). W.B. Saunders, Philadelphia, pp. 1531–1535 (1992)

Brain tumours. In *Forfar and Arneil's Textbook of Paediatrics*, 4th edn, Campbell A.G.M., McIntosh N. (eds). Churchill Livingstone, London, pp. 970–977 (1992)

KADOTA R.P., ALLEN J.B., HARTMAN G.A. and SPRUCE W.E. Brain tumours in children. *Journal of Pediatrics*, **114**, 511–519 (1989)

RORKE L.B., GILES F.H., DAVIS R.L. and BECKER L.E. Revision of the World Health Organisation classification of brain tumours for children. *British Journal of Cancer*, **56**, 1869–1886 (1985)

Case 54

Answers

Score

1. Acute retrocaecal appendicitis.
(+10)

Others

Q1: Appendicitis (+7).

(Easy)

Discussion

The history of central abdominal pain migrating to the right side of the abdomen is classical for acute appendicitis. The lack of abnormal signs on clinical examination may have been rather unusual – but then a retrocaecal appendix (which is what this boy had!) may not manifest as tenderness and guarding in the right iliac fossa. Flexion of the right lower limb alleviates the discomfort due to

138

the irritation of the nearby psoas muscle. A per rectum examination may well have clinched the diagnosis at the first visit. However, this is not a routine or recommended procedure in patients who may be immunocompromised, due to the risks associated with the resultant bacteraemia. Vincristine is associated with a neuropathy which can result in abdominal pain due to the ensuing severe constipation and, occasionally, an ileus. Also steroids taken by mouth can cause abdominal pain as a result of gastric ulceration and occasionally gastrointestinal perforation. However, neither of these two drugs would adequately explain the history and examination.

Further reading

Appendicitis. In *Nelson Textbook of Pediatrics*, 14th edn, Behrman R.E. (ed). W.B. Saunders, Philadelphia, pp. 897–990 (1992)

Appendicitis. In *Forfar and Arneil's Textbook of Paediatrics*, 4th edn, Campbell A.G.M., McIntosh N. (eds). Churchill Livingstone, London, pp. 1868–1869 (1992)

BRENDER J.D., MARCUSE E.K., KOEPSELL T.D. and HATCH E.L. Childhood appendicitis: factors associated with perforation. *Pediatrics*, **76**, 301–306 (1985)

WILKENSEN R.H., BARTLETT R.H. and ERAKLIS A.J. Diagnosis of appendicitis in infancy. *American Journal of Disease in Childhood*, **118**, 687–690 (1969)

Case 55

Answers

		Score
1.	Dietary history;	(+2)
	family history (+1) and drug history (+1).	(+2)
2.	X-ray knees and wrists (+1); alkaline phosphatase level (+1);	
	serum iron (+0.5); total iron binding capacity (+0.5).	(+3)
3.	Rickets (+2) and iron deficiency (+1).	(+3)

(+10)

(Average)

Discussion

This baby had slightly delayed gross motor developmental milestones. Having managed to walk for 3 months he then refused to bear weight on the lower limbs. He eventually presented to hospital following an intercurrent gastrointestinal illness, and was noted to have swollen wrists as well as a microcytic, hypochromic anaemia, mild hypocalcaemia and marked hypophosphataemia. The latter two biochemical abnormalities occur in severe rickets. Further corroborative evidence would be a raised serum alkaline phosphatase level and radiological changes typical of rickets. In dietary deficiency of vitamin D there is impaired absorption of calcium. This tends to lower the serum calcium level and stimulates the release of parathyroid hormone, restoring the calcium to normal or near-normal levels. This occurs at the expense of phosphate loss in the urine resulting in hypophosphataemia. There is inadequate mineralization of bone, an increase in the overall bone turnover and a concomitant rise in the alkaline phosphatase level. Subsequent bony deformities result in craniotabes, greenstick fractures, an impairment in linear growth, rickety rosary, bowed legs, swollen wrists and knees. Marked hypotonia is also a feature of this condition and may result in a regression or a delay in the attainment of motor milestones. Rickets usually follows dietary deficiencies but it is also a feature of severe malabsorption, lack of sunlight, chronic renal failure, chronic hepatic disease and prolonged use of anticonvulsants.

Several conditions, many of them familial, may result in rickets. The serum levels of calcium, phosphate and alkaline phosphatase found with these conditions are shown in the table below:

	Calcium	Phosphate	Alkaline phosphatase
1. Vitamin D deficiency	N/L	L	H

2. Hypophosphataemia
    vitamin D resistant rickets
    dietary, malabsorption
    oncogenic, TPN
    proximal RTA (type II)
    Fanconi syndromes
	N	L	H

3. Renal osteodystrophy	N/L	H	H
4. Vitamin D dependant rickets	L	N/L	H
5. Hypophosphatasia	N	N	L

N = normal; L = low; H = high; RTA = renal tubular acidosis

140

Further reading

Rickets. In *Nelson Textbook of Pediatrics*, 14th edn, Behrman R.E. (ed). W.B. Saunders, Philadelphia, pp. 141–145 and 1748–1753 (1992)

Rickets. In *Forfar and Arneil's Textbook of Paediatrics*, 4th edn, Campbell A.G.M., McIntosh N. (eds). Churchill Livingstone, London, pp. 1268–1272 and 1279–1280 (1992)

REICHEL H., KOEFFLER H.P. and NORMAN A.W. The role of the vitamin D endocrine system in health and disease. *New England Journal of Medicine*, **320**, 980–991 (1989)

CHESNEY R.W. Requirements and upper limits of vitamin D intake in the term neonate, infant and older child. *Journal of Pediatrics*, **116**, 159–166 (1990)

Case 56

Answers

		Score
1.	Paradoxical changes in blood pressure.	(+2)
2.	A Mantoux test (+2); echocardiogram (+2).	(+4)
3.	Tuberculous constrictive pericarditis.	(+2)
4.	Operative pericardiectomy (+1); antituberculous cover (+1).	(+2)
		(+10)

Others

Q2: ECG (+1); pericardial biopsy (+1); fasting gastric washing for acid fast bacilli (+1); ESR (+0.5) and autoantibodies (+0.5).
Q3: Constrictive pericarditis (+1.5); pericarditis (+1).

(Hard)

Discussion

This child has fluid overload as manifest by ascites, pedal and pulmonary oedema. While the liver size is impressive, the liver function tests and ultrasound do not indicate an inherent abnormality, suggesting hepatomegaly due to congestion. The vital clue to making the correct diagnosis in this case is the variation in the jugular venous filling with respiration. Normally the venous return to the heart increases as the intrathoracic pressure falls with inspiration, and this results in a diminution in the jugular venous pressure (JVP). The opposite occurs if there is some impediment to venous return. This is the case in acute respiratory failure or with a decrease in the filling capacity of the heart as seen in constrictive pericarditis. With the latter there is a paradoxical elevation of the JVP on inspiration (Kussmaul sign) and pulsus paradoxus. In addition, chronic restriction to right-sided venous filling results in hepatic congestion with ascites and pedal oedema. Restriction to left-sided venous filling results in pulmonary venous congestion, manifest clinically as basal crepitations, increased incidence of chest infections and prominent vascular markings with Kerley B lines on the chest X-ray. Bilateral restriction to venous return occurs acutely with cardiac tamponade and chronically with constrictive pericarditis. The latter may follow an episode of trauma, malignant infiltration, mediastinal irradiation, acute purulent pericarditis and tuberculous pericarditis. In this case the hilar calcification on the chest X-ray would point toward the last of these possible predisposing diagnoses.

Further reading

Constrictive pericarditis. In *Nelson Textbook of Pediatrics*, 14th edn, Behrman R.E. (ed). W.B. Saunders, Philadelphia, pp. 1219–1220 (1992)

Constrictive pericarditis. In *Forfar and Arneil's Textbook of Paediatrics*, 4th edn, Campbell A.G.M., McIntosh N. (eds). Churchill Livingstone, London, pp. 706–707 and 1398 (1992)

NISHIMURA R.A., CONNOLLY D.C., PARKIN T.W. and STANSON A.W. Constrictive pericarditis: assessment of current diagnostic procedures. *Mayo Clinics Proceedings*, **60**, 397–401 (1985)

SINZOBAHAMVYA N. and IKEOGU M.O. Purulent pericarditis. *Archives of Disease in Childhood*, **62**, 696–699 (1987)

STRANG J.I.G., KAKAZA H.H.S., GIBSON D.G. *et al.* Controlled trial of prednisolone as adjuvant in treatment of tuberculous constrictive pericarditis in Transkei. *Lancet*, **ii**, 1418–1422 (1987)

142

Case 57

Answers

	Score
1. α_1-antitrypsin phenotype for PiZZ (+1); prothrombin time (+1); liver biopsy (+1).	(+3)
2. α_1-antitrypsin deficiency.	(+3)
3. Regular vitamins A, D, E, K (+1); adequate diet to ensure weight gain (+1); review with liver biopsy at 6 months (+1).	(+4)
	─────
	(+10)

Others

Q1: TORCHES screen (+0.5); thyroid function tests (+0.5).

Q2: Neonatal hepatitis (+2); hypothyroidism (+1); cystic fibrosis (+1); tyrosinaemia (+1); Zellweger's syndrome (+0.5); Alagille syndrome (+0.5).

(Average)

Discussion

This baby, though otherwise well, presented with cholestatic jaundice after the first week of life. The physical examination showed mild icterus and a palpable liver. Investigation confirmed a mild elevation in liver enzymes and slow uptake and excretion of isotope on scintigraphy. The isotope managed to pass into the duodenum making biliary atresia (and other congenital causes of biliary tract obstruction) an unlikely diagnosis. Familial unconjugated hyperbilirubinaemia (Crigler–Najjar syndrome) generally presents with unremitting jaundice from day 2 or 3 of life and is associated with a high morbidity and risk of kernicterus. Inherited conjugated hyperbilirubinaemias (Dubin–Johnson and Rotor syndromes) produce mild icterus and rarely present before adolescence. The differential diagnosis in this case is therefore that of neonatal hepatitis due to an idiopathic, infective or metabolic cause. The infecting organisms include toxoplasmosis, rubella, CMV, herpes, hepatitis and entero viruses, syphilis and listeria. However, this baby was generally well and a serious congenital infection is

143

therefore unlikely. Metabolic causes include galactosaemia (unlikely without reducing substances in the urine), tyrosinaemia (amino acid profile was normal), cystic fibrosis (IRT was normal), Zellweger's syndrome (associated with hypotonia, retardation and abnormal facies), Alagille's syndrome (associated with abnormal facies, cardiac and vertebral anomalies), hypothyroidism and α_1-antitrypsin deficiency. Congenital hypothyroidism is associated with late onset jaundice but it is an unlikely diagnosis in an active baby who is feeding well. Therefore, in this case, α_1-antitrypsin deficiency is the 'best fit' diagnosis. In this condition there is a defective protease inhibitor (Pi). It is an autosomal recessive condition, acquired if both alleles result in the PiZZ phenotype (compared to the normal PiMM). The liver biopsy in affected individuals shows oedema and proliferation of bile ducts, cholestasis, piecemeal necrosis, periportal fibrosis and cellular inflammation. The severity of liver damage varies widely and can be assessed by repeating the liver biopsy after a few months. Management involves providing adequate nutrition and fat soluble vitamins. Currently, liver transplantation offers the best chance of long-term survival for these patients.

Further reading

α_1-antitrypsin deficiency. In *Nelson Textbook of Pediatrics*, 14th edn, Behrman R.E. (ed). W.B. Saunders, Philadelphia, pp. 1009–1017 (1992)

α_1-antitrypsin deficiency. In *Forfar and Arneil's Textbook of Paediatrics*, 4th edn, Campbell A.G.M., McIntosh N. (eds). Churchill Livingstone, London, pp. 651 and 1250 (1992)

BALISTRERI W.F. Neonatal cholestasis. *Journal of Pediatrics*, **106,** 171–184 (1985)

CRYSTAL R.G. α_1-antitrypsin deficiency, emphysema, and liver disease: genetic basis and strategies for therapy. *Journal of Clinical Investigation*, **85,** 1343–1352 (1990)

ABBOTT C.M., MCMAHON C.J., WHITEHOUSE D.B. and POVEY S. Prenatal diagnosis of α_1-antitrypsin deficiency using polymerase chain reaction. *Lancet*, **i,** 763–764 (1988)

Case 58

Answers

		Score
1.	Laron dwarfism (growth hormone insensitivity).	(+6)
2.	Insulin-like growth factors (IGF).	(+4)
		(+10)

Others

Q1: Russel-Silver dwarfism (+2), hypo/achondroplasia (+2); short
limbed dwarf (+1).

(Hard)

Discussion

This girl was extremely short, well below the 3rd centile, and had no
evidence of chronic illness, physical or mental abnormality. While
she maintained a normal growth velocity, she failed to respond to an
adequate course of growth hormone. This suggests that she has an
end-organ receptor insensitivity to growth hormone. This is confirmed by the investigations which showed elevated levels of
circulating growth hormone. This situation has been described in
children with Laron dwarfism. These children may have a small
nose with a depressed nasal bridge, a prominent forehead, obesity
and delayed but normal sexual maturation. The bone age is delayed
in most patients with Laron syndrome, though to a lesser degree
than the reduction in height for the chronological age. They have
high levels of growth hormone and growth hormone releasing
hormone, with low levels of insulin-like growth factors (e.g. IGF-1)
and those binding proteins which are growth hormone dependent
(e.g. IGFBP-3). This condition may be due to a deletion or a point
mutation in the growth hormone-binding receptor gene, and is
inherited in an autosomal recessive manner. Synthetic IGF-1
replacement has been given to some of these patients with
encouraging results. The preparation is given by regular subcutaneous injection and, because of its insulin-like properties, its use
may be complicated by hypoglycaemia.

Further reading

Laron dwarfism. In *Nelson Textbook of Pediatrics*, 14th edn, Behrman R.E. (ed). W.B.
    Saunders, Philadelphia, pp. 1400 (1992)
Laron dwarfism. In *Forfar and Arneil's Textbook of Paediatrics*, 4th edn, Campbell
    A.G.M., McIntosh N. (eds). Churchill Livingstone, London, pp. 1094 (1992)
LARON Z., PERTZELAN A. and MANNHEIMER S. Genetic pituitary dwarfism with high serum
    concentration of growth hormone. A new inborn error of metabolism? *Israel
    Journal of Medical Sciences*, **2**, 152–155 (1966)
ELDERS M.J., GARLAND J.T., DAUGHADAY W.A. *et al* Laron's dwarfism: studies on the nature of the
    defect. *Journal of Pediatrics*, **83**, 253–263 (1973)

LARON Z.V.I. An update on Laron syndrome. *Archives of Disease in Childhood*, **68**, 345–346 (1993)

LARON Z., LILOS P. and KLINGER B. Growth curves for Laron syndrome. *Archives of Disease in Childhood*, **68**, 768–770 (1993)

SAVAGE M.O., BLUM W.F., RANKE M.B. *et al* Clinical features and endocrine status in patients with growth hormone insensitivity (Laron syndrome). *Journal of Clinical Endocrinology and Metabolism*, **77**, 1465–1471 (1993)

Case 59

Answers

		Score
1.	Platelet count or full blood count.	(+5)
2.	Idiopathic thrombocytopenic purpura.	(+5)
		(+10)

Others

Q1: Bone marrow aspirate (+2); platelet antibodies (+1).
Q2: Acute leukaemia (+2).

(Easy)

Discussion

This child had a preceding viral illness, followed by an acute onset of bruises and petechiae. Generalized petechiae argues against non-accidental injury and implies the presence of thrombocytopenia or thrombopathia. Similarly the absence of pallor and generalized lymphadenopathy suggest that bone marrow failure due to an infiltrative process such as leukaemia is unlikely. Indeed, the most common diagnosis to present with this clinical scenario is idiopathic thrombocytopenic purpura (ITP). ITP occurs in 4 out of every 100 000 children, although the diagnosis is probably not made in several cases with minor symptoms. The outlook is generally excellent with full recovery of the platelet count within 3–6 months in 75% of patients. The mortality is less than 0.5% and this is usually due to intracranial bleeding, particularly during the first few weeks of the illness. In 70% of cases the problem usually follows an upper

146

respiratory tract infection which may act as the trigger whereby an immune process results in the development of platelet antibodies. The presenting platelet count is generally less than $20 \times 10^9/l$, the bleeding time is prolonged, and a bone marrow aspirate would show a normal or increased number of megakaryocytes. Many patients do not require treatment. However, most physicians would treat those patients with mucosal, fundal or gastrointestinal bleeding with a short course of prednisolone (1–2 mg/kg/day). Intravenous immunoglobulin can be given to those with life threatening bleeding not responsive to steroids.

Further reading

Idiopathic thrombocytopenic purpura. In *Nelson Textbook of Pediatrics*, 14th edn, Behrman R.E. (ed). W.B. Saunders, Philadelphia, pp. 1281–1282 (1992)

Idiopathic thrombocytopenic purpura. In *Forfar and Arneil's Textbook of Paediatrics*, 4th edn, Campbell A.G.M., McIntosh N. (eds). Churchill Livingstone, London, pp. 948–950 (1992)

BUCHANAN G.R. Childhood acute idiopathic thrombocytopenic purpura: How many tests and how much treatment required? *Journal of Pediatrics*, **106**, 928–930 (1985)

HALPERIN D.S. and DOYLE J.J. Is bone marrow examination justified in idiopathic thrombocytopenic purpura? *American Journal of Disease in Childhood*, **142**, 508–511 (1988)

MURPHY M.F., BROZOVIC B., MURPHY W., OUWEHAND W. and WATERS A.H. Guidelines for platelet transfusion. *Transfusion Medicine*, **2**, 311–318 (1992)

LILLEYMAN J.S. Idiopathic thrombocytopenic purpura: Where do we stand? *Archives of Disease in Childhood*, **59**, 701–703 (1984)

EDEN O.B. and LILLEYMAN J.S. (on behalf of the British Paediatric Haematology Group). Guidelines for management of idiopathic thrombocytopenic purpura. *Archives of Disease in Childhood*, **67**, 1056–1058 (1992)

Case 60

Answers

		Score
1.	Antihypertensives and anticonvulsants.	(+3)
2.	Doppler ultrasound renal arteries;	(+2)
	resting serum renin (+1), aortography (+1),	
	selective renal angiography (+1).	(+3)
3.	Renal artery stenosis.	(+2)
		(+10)

Others

Q2: Echocardiogram (+1); abdominal ultrasound (+1); ECG (+0.5); cardiac angiography (+0.5).

(Average)

Discussion

This boy had significant hypertension and a murmur. In such a case, coarctation of the aorta is a possibility. However, in coarctation of the aorta the systiolic blood pressure in the lower limbs is at least 20 mmHg lower than in the right upper limb (indeed, the blood pressure in the lower limbs was also raised!). Furthermore, the murmur is not typical of coarctation as it is not sited predominantly over the base of the heart and does not radiate to the left chest and back. In a child of this age with a coarctation one would also expect continuous murmurs over the upper back due to flow in collateral vessels. The systolic murmur was, in fact, heard best over the abdomen. Although abdominal coarctation does occur, this condition is also associated with diminished pulses and a lowered blood pressure in the lower limbs. In contrast, stenosis of the renal artery would result in a harsh systolic bruit heard best over the abdomen and systemic hypertension.

Further reading

Hypertension and renal artery stenosis. In *Nelson Textbook of Pediatrics*, 14th edn, Behrman R.E. (ed). W.B. Saunders, Philadelphia, pp. 1222–1227 (1992)

Hypertension and renal artery stenosis. In *Forfar and Arneil's Textbook of Paediatrics*, 4th edn, Campbell A.G.M., McIntosh N. (eds). Churchill Livingstone, London, pp. 707–709 (1992)

Report of the Second Task Force on blood pressure control in children. *Pediatrics,* **79,** 1–25 (1987)

LOGGIE J.M.H. Hypertension in children and adolescents: Causes and diagnostic studies. *Journal of Pediatrics,* **74,** 331–355 (1969)

DEAL J.E., BARRATT T.M. and DILLON M.J. Management of hypertensive emergencies. *Archives of Disease in Childhood,* **67,** 1089–1092 (1992)

List of normal values

Sample	Children	Neonates
Chemical pathology		
Blood		
Sugar (fasting)	3.3–5.5 mmol/l	2.2–4.4 mmol/l
Blood ammonia	21–47 μmol/l	34–107 μmol/l
Plasma		
Bicarbonate	21–25 mmol/l	18–23 mmol/l
Chloride	95–106 mmol/l	–
Creatinine	0.02–0.08 mmol/l	0.02–0.1 mmol/l
Potassium	3.5–5.6 mmol/l	4.3–7.6 mmol/l
Sodium	135–145 mmol/l	132–145 mmol/l
Urea	2.5–6.6 mmol/l	–
Serum		
Acid phosphatase	5.0–12.6 U/l	7.4–19.4 U/l
Albumin	34–48 g/l	25–55 g/l
α-Fetoprotein	<15 U/ml	<55,000 U/ml
α_1-Antitrypsin	1.8–4.0 g/l	1.5–4.0 g/l
ALT	10–40 U/l	10–80 U/l
Alkaline phosphatase	100–850 U/l	<1,500 U/l
Amylase	100–400 U/l	<50 U/l
AST	10–45 U/l	10–75 U/l
Bilirubin (total)	1.7–26 μ mol/l	<205 μ mol/l
Calcium	2.20–2.75 mmol/l	1.85–3.05 mmol/l
Cholesterol	3.1–6.8 mmol/l	2.4–5.6 mmol/l
CPK	8.0–60 U/l	30–300 U/l
Ferritin	10–100 ng/ml	100–500 ng/ml
Folic acid	11–34 nmol/l	15–40 nmol/l
γGT	5–32 U/l	13–147 U/l
IgA	0.3–3.0 g/l	0.0–0.08 g/l
IgG	5.0–15 g/l	6.3–17 g/l
IgM	0.4–2.0 g/l	0.0–0.2 g/l
Iron	10.7–31.3 μmol/l	19.7–48.3 μmol/l
Iron binding capacity	45–72 μmol/l	11–31 μmol/l
LDH	58–230 U/l	325–1825 U/l
Lead	<1.9 μmol/l	–
Magnesium	0.6–0.95 mmol/l	0.58–1.0 mmol/l
Osmolality	275–295 mmol/kg H_2O	260–300 mmol/kg H_2O
Phosphate	1.16–1.91 mmol/l	1.58–2.87 mmol/l
Protein	62–80 g/l	46–77 g/l
Uric acid	0.12–0.42 mmol/l	12–50 mmol/l
Urine		
Calcium	750–3,750 μmol/24 h	<1,000 μmol/24 h
Ca^{2+}: creatinine ratio	<0.7 mmol/mmol	–
Chloride	<4.0 mmol/kg/24 h	1.3–3.3 mmol/kg/24 h

Sample	Children	Neonates
Creatinine	44–354 μmol/kg/24 h	88–176 μmol/kg/24 h
Creatinine clearance	95–150 ml/min/1.73 m^2	40–65 ml/min/1.73 m^2
pH	5.3–7.2	>5
Phosphate	15–20 mg/kg/24 h	<200 mg/24 h
Potassium	<2.0 mmol/kg/24 h	<2.3 mmol/kg/24 h
Protein	30–50 mg/24 h	<10 mg/24 h
Sodium	<3.7 mmol/kg/24 h	<4.4 mmol/kg/24 h
Urea	150–600 mmol/24 h	2.5–4.5 mmol/24 h
Urea clearance	50–90 ml/min/1.73 m^2	–
Uric acid	3.0–12 mmol/24 h	–
Haematology		
Fibrinogen	5.8–11.6 μmol/l	4.4–10.3 μmol/l
FDP	12.3–19.5 mg/l	–
Haemoglobin	10.5–14 g/dl	13–20 g/dl
Haematocrit	33–42%	42–66%
MCH	24–30 pg	32–40 pg
MCHC	30–36 g/dl	34–36 g/dl
MCV	76–88 fl	86–106 fl
Platelets	150–450 × 10^9/l	100–300 × 10^9/l
Red cells	3.5–5.6 × 10^{12}/l	4–5.8 × 10^{12}/l
White cells	5–21 × 10^9/l	6–15 × 10^9/l
eosinophils	2–3%	3%
lymphocytes	51%	48%
monocytes	4–8%	6–12%
neutrophils	32–52%	30–50%
reticulocytes	0–2%	0–2%
CSF		
Red cells	0–2 × 10^6/l	0–675 × 10^6/l
White cells	0–10 × 10^6/l	0–14 × 10^6/l
Protein	200–400 mg/l	250–900 mg/l
Sugar	2.8–4.4 mmol/l	–
Arterial blood gas		
Po$_2$	11.3–14 kPa	9.3–13.3 kPa
Pco$_2$	4.7–6.0 kPa	–
pH	7.35–7.42	–
Base excess	2.5 to −2.5 mmol/l	−2.5 mmol/l
Hormone levels		
Cortisol (0800 h)	200–720 nmol/l	330–1,700 nmol/l

Sample	Children	Neonates
Cortisol (2400 h)	<205 nmol/l	–
FSH	<3.0 U/l (prepuberty)	–
GH (basal)	<5 mU/l	–
GH (peak)	>15 mU/l	–
Luteinising hormone	<1.9 U/l (prepuberty)	–
Oestradiol	<70 μmol/l (prepuberty)	–
Testosterone	<3.5 nmol/l (prepuberty)	–
Testosterone	10–30 nmol/l (puberty)	–
Thyroxine	70–180 nmol/l	75–350 nmol/l
TSH	0.3–5 mU/l	<10 mU/l
17-ketosteroids	–	<2.5 mg/24 h
17-OH progesterone	<14 mmol/l	<30 mmol/l
Miscellaneous		
72 h faecal fat	<2 g/24 h	–
1 h serum xylose	>1.13 mmol/l (after 5 g oral dose)	–

Centile charts

GIRLS: BIRTH – 18 YEARS; HEIGHT CENTILES

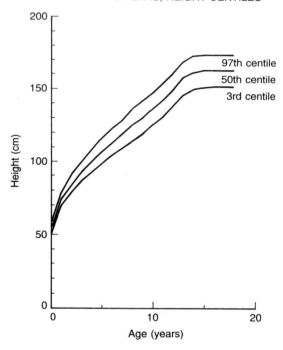

GIRLS: BIRTH – 18 YEARS; WEIGHT CENTILES

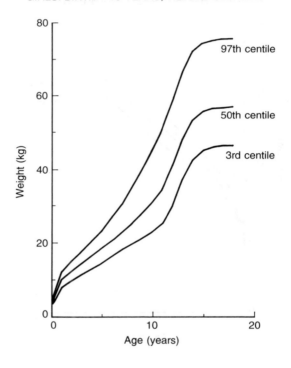

Index